João Costa
Health as a Social System

Health, Communication and Society | Volume 4

To my grandson Vincent

João Costa is a public health specialist and health economist. He has a doctorate degree from the London School of Hygiene and Tropical Medicine. He has around 40 years of work experience in development projects aiming at strengthening health systems in several countries. His professional and contractual relations included links with academic institutions, consultancy companies, international development banks, international development agencies, and others. Currently, he works as independent consultant.

João Costa
Health as a Social System
Luhmann's Theory Applied to Health Systems. An Introduction

[transcript]

Diese Publikation wurde im Rahmen des Fördervorhabens 16TOA002 mit Mitteln des Bundesministeriums für Bildung und Forschung im Open Access bereitgestellt.

Bibliographic information published by the Deutsche Nationalbibliothek
The Deutsche Nationalbibliothek lists this publication in the Deutsche Nationalbibliografie; detailed bibliographic data are available in the Internet at http://dnb.d-nb.de

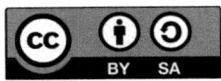

This work is licensed under the Creative Commons Attribution-ShareAlike 4.0 (BY-SA) which means that the text may be remixed, build upon and be distributed, provided credit is given to the author and that copies or adaptations of the work are released under the same or similar license.
Creative Commons license terms for re-use do not apply to any content (such as graphs, figures, photos, excerpts, etc.) not original to the Open Access publication and further permission may be required from the rights holder. The obligation to research and clear permission lies solely with the party re-using the material.

First published in 2023 by transcript Verlag, Bielefeld
© **João Costa**

Cover layout: Maria Arndt, Bielefeld
Cover illustration: João Costa
Printed by: Majuskel Medienproduktion GmbH, Wetzlar
https://doi.org/10.14361/9783839466933
Print-ISBN 978-3-8376-6693-9
PDF-ISBN 978-3-8394-6693-3
ISSN of series: 2940-1828
eISSN of series: 2940-1836

Printed on permanent acid-free text paper.

Contents

Presentation 7

Introduction 11

Chapter 1 – Niklas Luhmann's Social Systems Theory – Concepts 27

Chapter 2 – General application of the theory 53

Chapter 3 – Health Systems – Methodological issues 63

Chapter 4 – Health Systems Thinking and Social Systems Theory 69

Chapter 5 – Health Systems Thinking Tools and Social Systems Theory 81

Chapter 6 – Health Systems Strengthening and Systems Theory 107

Chapter 7 – Health Organizations and Poly-contexturality 121

Chapter 8 – Critics' Views about Luhmann's Theory 129

Chapter 9 – Prospects and Examples 139

Final Remarks – Science or Technology 165

References 171

Annex – Advanced Topics 181

Presentation

This book has two aims: first, to introduce Niklas Luhmann's Social Systems Theory to students and researchers of health systems interested in health services provision as a social system; second, to encourage the use of Luhmann's theory in health systems research. During his productive life, Luhmann covered the social systems of media, law, politics, economy, art, education, religion and others. However, he did not apply his theory to health as comprehensively as he did for the other systems. This book therefore is an attempt to apply his concepts more extensively to health services provision and show the analytical possibilities the theory opens.

In the international health arena, Health Systems Strengthening (HSS) and Health Systems Thinking (HST) have acquired prominence, influencing agendas of international organizations and academic institutions in the last two decades. However, the theoretical underpinning is sketchy, borrowing concepts and tools from diverse fields of knowledge, without a unifying vision of what a health system is. Although it has received some attention, Luhmann's theory is largely unknown among health researchers, and the resources the theory provides for solving identified weaknesses remain untapped. The Social Systems Theory constitutes an integrated theoretical body with consistent articulation of a number of constructs; therefore it has more to offer than just collections of unrelated theories and narrow frameworks.

Luhmann's theory is complex and has a plethora of concepts. It was developed over the course of around 30 years. This book has been conceived to introduce a comprehensive summary of the theory for those who are coming into contact with Luhmann's work for the first time or have only superficial information about it. Therefore, the text tries to be as reader-friendly as is possible for such a conceptually rich theory. Nevertheless, the book also introduces references to advanced topics for those interested in delving deeper into the theory.

The book is structured with an introduction and nine chapters. The chapters intend to gradually immerse the reader in the conceptual network while acquiring a good grasp of its particularities. With this orientation, the **introduction** prepares the ground for the subsequent discussions, presenting the current use of notions of systems in health systems studies.

The **Chapter 1** presents the key concepts of the theory. **Chapter 2** applies the concepts to health systems, referring to the texts Luhmann wrote on health as a social system, where he stated that the systems of provision of healthcare could be analysed as a social system, having standard features of functional social systems. This chapter is a generic application of the theory with brief explanations about how the theoretical concepts can explain health systems' structural and functional features, without looking into details of programmes, institutional roles and operations.

Chapter 3 discusses methodological issues concerning research within the scope of the theory and **Chapter 4** discusses the differences between health system from Luhmann's perspective and Health Systems Thinking (HST) approaches. This chapter discusses critical views of HST. Sequentially, in light of the theory, **Chapter 5** offers in-depth discussions of tools promoted by HST.

Chapter 6 further expands the application of the theory and presents *methodological* implications for *health systems strengthening* initiatives; it introduces the discussion of relations between *political systems* and health systems; and discusses issues of *complexity* and health systems. The chapter reflects on important implications for applications of the theory.

Chapter 7 is dedicated to *health organizations*, such as hospitals and polyclinics. Occupying a prominent position in Luhmann's conceptual architecture, organizations are defined as one of the three types of social system. His theoretical contributions in the field of management theory have received considerable attention in Scandinavian and German-speaking countries. Health systems researchers may find valuable elements for reflection.

Chapter 8 presents some criticisms that have been formulated about Luhmann's theory. Readers interested in becoming further acquainted with the debates will find the pertinent literature recommended in the chapter. **Chapter 9** reflects on the way forward, exploring possible avenues for applications of the theory, discussing a number of alternative approaches and interpretations of recently published health systems research.

Final remarks addresses the issue of assessing theories, distinguishing science from the technologies it brings about. The message is directed to those interested in reflecting on the value of the work of building and assembling theories.

An **Annex** is added to introduce some advanced topics; readers can find snapshots of the more demanding conceptualizations appearing in Luhmann's works, such as: Medium and forms; Symbolically generalized medium of communication; Paradoxes and contingency formulas; Structural features of the political system.

While readers may have interest in the topics addressed in specific chapters, it would be advisable to start with the introduction and the first two chapters, and move on to selecting the theme of interest. The composition of the chapters follow an ascendant "spiral" format, whereby the theoretical concepts reappear, progressively bringing formulations of higher levels of complexity.

Due to author's limitations, Luhmann's original texts in German could not be studied. However, readers will find in the reference section an extensive list of Luhmann's books published in English and Spanish, with a number of Luhmann's key texts that are not found in English but are available in Spanish translation.

Introduction

Preliminary discussion

Let's start with the basic concept, the notion of system itself. There were and still are countless definitions of "system". We do not list them here or try a comprehensive categorization of those notions. For our purpose at this point, we only need reflect on what a system is. That is the question: what is a system?

The first answer that may come to our minds is a unit. When something is called a system, the notion of unit is immediately conveyed; a unit with collections of elements inside; a sort of a set in mathematic terms, whose elements have relations among themselves.

With this notion comes the corollary idea of limits and, with that, the abstract image of internal and external difference, in whatever conceptual space we may project it. Thus, something belongs to the system while something else doesn't. The opposition can be characterized as a distinction between system and environment. Some things belong to the system and everything else to the environment, including other systems that may exist there.

The acceptance of this apparently trivial distinction between system and environment paves the way to additional considerations. There must be something that regulates the borders, to use an appealing metaphor. There must be mechanisms, processes, and rules, or whatever we may call it, that does the job of selecting what to "let" in while the rest remains outside.

We can then imagine that this active process is carried out by regulatory instances of the system itself. But we can also imagine that something we may call "system" does not have any such selective capability. A new distinction we may make here then is that the so-called self-referenced system carries out the selections while the other type doesn't.

Self-reference therefore implies an active way of selecting. In whatever way it might be done, in correspondence with some sort of "self-identity", some systems are able to perform such an operation as opposed to others without such "refinement", as we could call it.

In the first case, the observer is the system itself; in the other case, the observer is outside it, drawing borders and defining the content and limits of the system – being the system, a construction of that external observer. Yes, we have brought the figure of the observer into our considerations. It is necessary to recognize that observations are being carried out, and they play a role in the constitution of systems.

It seems that we now have two clear categories of systems, those that self-regulate and those that do not have any such functionality, in spite of the ordered functions they may display. Surely the two types are still mental representations of phenomena we observe. However, we accept that those capable of self-regulation are endowed with aims that, in contrast, the others are not.

Let's get into some more concrete examples. A planetary system does not seem to have any self-regulated selection competence.[1] Whatever is pulled by gravitational forces may be incorporated into the planetary system without any determinant other than mass and speed.

Likewise, an ecological system does not seem to conduct any selection of the species living in it. A large piece of land can have a number of species on it and they can, theoretically, at some point in time, all be replaced by other species and the ecological system will remain as such. An ecological system does not show preferences.

What would destroy those systems (the ecological and the planetary) is not error or failures in what should be brought in and kept in or left out. They can be destroyed by the annihilation of their limits. On the other hand, there are different types of system that, although equally destructible by obliteration of their limits, need to be rigorous in their selection of what belongs to it and what does not.

We can say that social systems are indeed that sort of system. They need constantly to keep deploying their selection criteria. Let's think, for instance, of a health system. If we accept that health systems are indeed social systems, and this is an important decision with many implications, we can see that this is a self-referential system, dealing with matters that are its concern.

A health system would not be concerned with issues that belong to, for instance, the legal system – another social system. The complexities of legal def-

---

1   Unless one adopts the idea that gravity fulfils that role, implying the principle that gravity has a deliberative function, which no physicist has so far attempted to describe.

initions, interpretation and argumentation are alien to the health system and vice versa. Judges and lawyers often resort to technical medical opinion, but the rationale and construction of the medical expert's argument would not be a matter of legal scrutiny. The expert conclusion is enough from the legal perspective.

Likewise, the health expert would not be troubled by what the legal professionals do with their expert opinions as the intricacies of the legal interpretation is beyond their realm. In these two cases, the legal system and the health system need to maintain the regulatory mechanisms that perform the selection of themes and topics that are matters of concern for them.

Health professionals are highly sensitive to any medical opinion without the identifiable marks of a legitimate medical communication. Impostors can be easily identified. They do not belong to the system, nor do their communications. We have here a key word: communication.

We can anticipate here that these lines of argumentation reflect Niklas Luhmann's comprehensive theory of Social Systems that this book is about. There will be a lot more about him in the chapters to come. For the moment, we can say that Luhmann categorically said that the only thing that is capable of building social systems is communication. "A social systems emerges when communication develops from communication" (Luhmann 2013, p. 53). This statement may be a tough one to begin with, but its corollary – any social system would cease to exist if its respective communications no longer happened – is easier to assimilate.

So, when we talk about systems' limits, and in particular social systems' limits, we talk about the universe of semantics that make the communication inside the system meaningful in itself. And, it is important to emphasize, "meaningful to itself", regardless of outsiders' views. This is how social systems' limits are drawn.

The selections made at the borders of a social system carries out the "triage" of communications, with recognizable meanings therefore allowed to circulate internally. Only the system can control what belongs to it or not; no other system can perform such operations for any other social system. Otherwise the borders and the system itself would be destroyed.

We can try to wrap this up by saying: yes, health is a system; yes, it is a social system; it can control what belongs to it (or does not); this self-reference keeps it differentiated from everything else in its environment; only the health system can perform the operations it recognizes as its, and no other system can do that for the health system. It is impossible to downplay the relevance of these assertions. There will be a lot more about these themes throughout the following pages. For the moment, though, we can go to our brief historical review.

Health Systems – main approaches

Strong awareness of the systemic character of healthcare service provision emerged by the end of the twentieth century. The structures and organizations of health services started to be considered as having characteristics of systems. Around the same time, departments and units focusing on health systems studies started to appear in universities around the Globe, and diverse notions of systems were brought into debates.

From the acknowledgement of health sectors' systemic features, countless studies and concepts have been deployed, establishing health systems as an important research topic and target for development aid. A key moment for the establishment of the topic was the WHO's *World Health Report* (Health Systems: Improving Performance – WHO 2000), and years later the proposition of the Six Building Blocks (six pillars) framework (WHO 2007).

The trend grew stronger with the promotion and dissemination of guidance for health systems strengthening by international organizations and development agencies, alongside the establishment of health systems thinking approaches also fully supported by the WHO, with the publication of *Systems Thinking for Health Systems Strengthening* (WHO 2009).

This book extensively discusses these references in light of Social Systems Theory. The usefulness and relevance of those views about health systems cannot be underestimated, and their appearance in the international health arena has significantly marked the orientation in addressing public health problems.

Nevertheless, this book also points to their weaknesses, particularly originating from the lack of a clear understanding of social systems. The Six Pillars framework is discussed in the next section and the other two major references, health systems strengthening and health systems thinking are respectively discussed in specific subsequent chapters.

Key STEP - WHO Six Pillars framework

The health systems six building blocks (the six pillars) framework promoted by the World Health Organization (WHO, 2007) has become a major influence for health systems research since its publication. Subsequent works, broadly linked to health systems thinking (WHO, 2009), added other concepts, tools and references imported from a range of different sources from social science to general systems theories.

Concurrently, major agencies supporting health systems in development aid contexts, including the Global Fund for Fighting AIDS, Tuberculosis and Malaria, GAVI (The Vaccine Alliance), World Bank, and bilateral agencies such as the British DfID (Department for International Development), the American USAID (United States Agency for International Development), the German GIZ (Gesellschaft für Internationale Zusammenarbeit), and others, published their views on this key issue, Health Systems Strengthening, which is strongly influenced by the WHO Six Pillars framework. The conceptual field of international health is very much constructed by the works, now comprehensively addressed under the banner of "Health Systems Thinking".

The Six Pillars framework is based on simple notions of systems as comprising articulated parts, whereby changes in one component have effects on the others. In this section we discuss the evident purpose of the Six Pillars framework to assist developing countries as well as development aid donors in the early twenty-first century context to reflect on the systemic nature of health systems.

The framework calls for cautious assessment of system-wide implications of any investment in the health sector, taking into account that massive injection of resources in some projects and programmes can have powerful distorting effects on everything else, undermining the capacity of the recipient health system to respond adequately to its on-going challenges.

However, it has become clear that the framework has limitations for comprehensive analyses of health systems structures and dynamics, particularly for analysing health systems in more complex settings, in developing as well as developed countries. The subsequent attempts to bring systems analysis to a higher conceptual ground, although enriching the conceptual arsenal, did not achieve the desired consistency, as pointed out in widely read papers such as Balabanova et al. (2010), which have repeatedly asked for more studies on the theoretical background of systems research.

It may sound ironic that high-profile academic experts, who were themselves expected to propose solutions for the weaknesses they pointed out, were in fact only asking for more studies and more contributions. Evidently, they did not know where to find the answers they were looking for.

The banner itself, "Health Systems Thinking", rather conveys the message that this is a field where questions instead of answers predominate. There is also a certain irony in a field of knowledge being named and defined by the basic method of approaching any topic – "thinking". In the history of scientific knowledge there may not be any field defined in such a way. Thinking is surely the basic process for pursuing knowledge on anything; this is self-evident. Therefore, one cannot avoid the thought that such formulation reveals lack of option and the powerlessness of having no other way of conceptually addressing the subject called "health system". How do we deal with it? The answer seems to be: "we do not know, but we can carry on *thinking*".

Here we therefore suggest that some of this hopelessness derives from the weaknesses of the frameworks so far adopted. We focus on the Six Pillars framework in this introduction, as the succeeding currents – Health Strengthening and Health Systems Thinking – are dealt with in specific chapters of the book. After Luhmann's theory is presented in the first chapter, his concepts can then be used in the discussions of those two approaches.

For the discussion on the Six Pillars framework in this introduction, we do not use Luhmann's conceptual tools, as they are presented later, but our discussion is thoroughly informed by Luhmann's views on social systems. This introduction mainly focuses on the lack of systemic features in the notion of pillars and therefore the limited scope the framework offers for systems analysis.

Overview

The WHO's Six Pillars framework conceives health systems as comprised of the following components: medicines, vaccines and other technologies; health information; health service delivery; health workforce; leadership and governance; and financing.

Evidently these pillars are basic structural and functional features of any large healthcare services complex, with inpatient and outpatient facilities, and all related support. In principle, the Six Pillars structure intends to portray a macro-level, nationwide institutional apparatus, commonly viewed as comprising ministries of health and/or related institutions, according to the political organization of the country's healthcare service provision. Nevertheless, the same pillar structures can be found as distinctive features of large providers of healthcare services, including diverse types of organizations, public and private alike. The intention behind the WHO formulation was, however, specifically orientated towards public systems or equivalent structures intended to serve the population of a country.

The idea of system informing this vision consists basically of the notion of an interconnected set of components, drawing from a limited pool of resources (human, financial, equipment, etc.), exchanging inputs between them and generating measurable outputs. The framework suggests the existence of central coordination of some sort, represented by the governance pillar, with support from the health information pillar.

This model comprehends a structural whole, where each part is relevant and affects all the others, and therefore depends on the others for its operations. The model portrays the system as being the unit that brings the individual pillars together, having dynamic pull that interlinks all parts.

An intrinsic modus operandi is understood to be at work in such a system, and planners, managers and researchers should account for all interconnectivity of the systemic parts. Unplanned, unforeseen and undesirable effects may spread across the system, in correspondence with its integrated characteristic. The framework therefore calls for comprehensive attention in any effort to change operations and functionalities of any elements of the pillars.

The framework came as a response to the growing concerns over the impact of specific aid programmes (Hafner and Shiffman, 2013), and drew attention when the inflow of supports to health systems in developing countries started to cause disruptions, with excess resources going into some programmes without a clear understanding of their systemic interrelationships.

The intention then was to create a tool for approaching health systems in their interconnectedness. Such a tool should guide the explorations to be carried out, focusing on the connections between the parts. Therefore, the model became an observational tool intended to generate descriptions of the constitution of the system, and to communicate those narratives in decision-making processes. The framework entertained the ambition that once health is properly understood in its systemic features, and therefore cautiously studied, interventions are more likely to succeed or, at least, prevent avoidable disruptions.

In conclusion, the Six Pillars framework is a tool for a health system to observe itself. It was made available for any health system to use it as a reference for self-observation. However good the intentions, another story was whether the tool was or was not properly employed; whether the tool delivered convincing arguments in the midst of the political struggles and decision-making dynamics.

On the face of it, a more comprehensive view of health systems has to account for the dynamics and systemic structural and functional dimensions where such tools are or are not used, and do or don't achieve the expected effects. In admitting such processes of tool selection and use, the self-observation capability of health systems comes to the fore and, with it, self-reference as a feature of the system and its components. This self-referential functionality was not considered within the Six Pillars framework. A more comprehensive framework is therefore needed to incorporate such complexities.

Furthermore, envisaging a comprehensive view of health systems that could be applied to any country context, developed and developing alike, the framework clearly represents a modest attempt to reduce the immense complexity and diversity of elements of any health system.

A comprehensive view of a health system must include: the regulatory functions of the professional bodies; the distinct role of public health within a system predominantly orientated to curative care; the large sets of programmes and interventions under the banner of health promotion, community health and health education of communities; the diversity of interest groups including patients' associations and advocacy; the institutional roles of entities assessing and issuing accreditation and quality certificates, etc.

Perhaps even more important, the understanding of health systems should account for the huge variety of autonomous components in the service delivery field as well as in the provision of inputs such as medicines, and how, despite their variety, they are distinctly and unquestionably part of the same health system. The notion of health systems informing an all-inclusive analysis needs to reflect the diversity of entities and their distinct modus operandi. The following sub-sections discuss in detail questions about structures and functionalities of the pillars.

Tracing decision-making in the pillars

The WHO's notion of pillar conveys the idea of integrated elements, assembled in distinct units whose operations are similar, possibly articulated and coherently brought together. But in the real world the outlook of the so-called pillars is of rather fragmented sets independently composed of several distinct and mostly unrelated entities. The pillars in fact do not constitute coordinated operational units covering all elements identified as belonging to the same pillar.

Taking, for example, the medicines pillar. Entities dealing with medicines appear in diverse organizational settings; they can be independent and autonomous sellers, wholesale operators, divisions inside hospitals, dispensers at Primary Health Care (PHC) facilities, etc. Medicines may be provided by public facilities under public funding arrangements, where patients can get them for free or for a small fee. In other cases, patients may have to pay out of their own pockets for most of the medicines they need, if they find them at private, regulated (or not) pharmacies. Patients could also be reimbursed for some drugs by health insurance arrangements they may be covered by. The variety as well as independence of the entities involved is usually large. At the same time, regulations on pharmaceuticals are ubiquitous and, in one way or another, all countries set rules for producing, importing, storing, assuring quality, commercializing, managing, prescribing and dispensing drugs. Although large variety can be expected among countries' willingness and capacity to adopt and enforce rules, the existence of rules is pervasive. However, on the operational side, much depends on what the organizations and entities in the system are capable of. Besides that, structural features, such as whether there are only private independent healthcare providers, or a mix of public and private ones, or only public ones, may have crucial influence on the overall aggregated "performance" of the pillar. In short, what is called the medicine pillar can hardly be seen as a consistent and coherent unit linked to the other pillars according to precise, simple and unique rules. In this regard, the notion of pillar gives a false impression of what actually goes on.

The same sort of fragmentation can also be observed in the way health information is gathered, analysed and used at several structural and functional levels of any health system. Health information management systems respond to a huge variety of purposes. The purpose can vary greatly. For instance, to give a few examples: operations in programmes such as referral of patients across PHC facilities; internal communication of operational services in large hospitals; gathering of nationwide vital statistics; regional epidemiological surveillance, etc. Each case has distinct concerns, and adopts independent diverse solutions. Not all information systems need to be under the same managerial and decision-making structure or be implemented across the board in all healthcare services providers under a unique nationwide organization.

Human resources pillars also cannot be seen as a sole entity. Besides the centralized management of, say, ministry of health staff, there are countless possibilities for human resources to be independently managed by the structures of service provision that exist in the country, such as private providers, charities, large autonomous public complexes. Each can have independent management and decision-making processes related to their own human resources.

Because of the large variety of component entities, and given the multiplicity of ways these components are set up and autonomously operate within the system, health systems constitute a considerable challenge for comprehensive application of the Six Pillars framework. The disposition of elements in the presumed pillars is multifaceted, rather than uniform and unique. Again, the diversity of configurations of structures and practices is oversimplified by the notion of pillars.

In short, the pillars, as conceived in the framework, are not organizations; they do not operate as such. The pillars are abstract collections of practices and resources without objective organizational expression, which makes them of very limited value for understanding the dynamics and complexities of health systems.

The centrality of services delivery

Healthcare services delivery is the core business of any health system; this may sound like stating the obvious and no further justification is required. However, the Six Pillars framework redirects the focus of attention to the set of pillars itself, without recognizing the crucial importance of communication in continuously building the system in sets of healthcare provision.

Approaching health service delivery as a pillar among others does not properly account for its centrality or its high level of complexity. In any country, health services are delivered by thousands of providers, with large variation of interdependences or independence. Regardless of the diversity, the delivery of healthcare services is central to the justification and reproduction of any organizations taken part in healthcare as a social function.

Service delivery cannot be considered only a pillar among others because it is essential and fundamental; without it there is no health system of any kind. The other pillars may even disappear for some time, or may not have existed historically, while the health system, or some proto-system in embryonic stage, was already functioning at the early stages of the historical development of health systems.² The other pillars appeared at later stages, mainly in connection with technological developments.

In situations of catastrophe or war, the systems may regress to those early precarious junctures where nothing else but the fundamental health communications among providers and between providers and patients still work. Someone recognized as a doctor by individuals or communities may communicate with patients about, for example, putting hot or cold compresses on the part of the body affected. That could be a healing technique stripped down to the bare minimum in circumstances that cannot offer any other option. Nevertheless, health messages are still communicated and accepted, and the authoritative roles find expression and sustain the structural fundamentals of the system. Once the temporary crises are over, from that rudimentary persistent base the system evolves into previous or even new complex articulations.

On the governance pillar

The question of fragmentation and diversity of components is relevant for understanding how governance operates and how little the notion of pillar helps to a good understanding of what goes on. A key issue concerns how distributed or concentrated are governance roles performed in a health system. If the governance pillar were thought of as a centralized command in charge of defining, regulating and deciding on all operations of all pillars, that would imply overstretching the pillar with a highly complex and impossible task of actually directing a huge variety of performances taking place in an equally huge range of settings.

These questions arise from the lack of definition in the framework of whether autonomy is or is not a relevant feature of the pillars. On one side, the pillars are not formulated as organized units and all the regulatory functions are supposed to be performed by the governance pillar. On the contrary, if the pillars are supposed to have some level of autonomous regulations and decision-making powers, that would empty the governance pillar of its key roles, and leave the overall coordination of the pillars to their own abilities, making the stability of the whole system less likely.

---

2   The works of Canguilhem (1978) and Foucault (2003) shed light on the constitution of healthcare services with systemic characteristics although these authors did not use such terminology. That discussion is beyond the scope of this section.

Therefore, the governance problem has to be solved at some intermediate level, where overarching rules might be defined centrally but decision-making capabilities should be distributed across the autonomous entities, as is for instance the case in autonomous hospitals, making decisions concerning all matters in all pillars. In short, the notion of pillars creates an insurmountable problem for mapping out and convening all the diverse regulatory, accountability and decision-making roles into a single governance pillar

Surely, a certain level of self-observation and self-management is carried out at each organization and respective divisions implementing the pillars' operations. For instance, the work carried out inside the health information sections (be it at ministerial, regional, organizational or facility level), is indeed the object of continuous self-evaluation by those working in those sections, wherever their location. Hospitals have their own health information system for their own management, to assess operational performances, optimizing routines and many more applications. The same can be said about the medicines pillar. Any pharmacy, whether inside or outside health facilities, autonomous, independent or subordinated to a network, has its own internal self-maintained processes for controlling storages, dispensing, purchasing, selling, etc.

The systemic nature and complexity of a health system implies necessary reliance on degrees of self-management competences at all levels and components. This brings to the fore the question on how every element in the system can act in accordance with what needs to be done at whatever level the element is located, no matter the linkages with other elements in the system. In other words, governance becomes a matter of alignment (where necessary) of the operations of all of a system's components with the orientation of the overarching system they belong to. Governance therefore has to become a reality in a context of internal differentiation of the system, where the components should have autonomous status.

In this sense, it is impossible to conceive of coordination of distributed competences without organizations performing their decision roles within their structures and functions. The argument can also be presented in the following terms: if socially relevant decisions are being made, they belong to the organization, where those decisions are communicated to the respective members and those affected by it. In consequence, we can say that the pillars do not make decisions; decisions are made by the organizations that can be conceptually described as being linked to one pillar or another, but the pillars themselves are not organizations, and therefore do not have the features and functionalities of organizations.

The distribution of decision-making capabilities across all organizations in the health system (no matter the pillar) raises pertinent questions about the capacity of the organizations to correspond and comply with the applicable orientations emanating from core regulatory bodies of the health system. However, every organization is still individually concerned with operational and "survival" matters, about which they are the sole responsible decision-makers.

Health systems' governance structures and self-regulatory mechanisms

If the reflections in the previous section are valid, the model of governance to achieve a systemic dynamism is not one of a unified command structure with subordination of the whole system to a centralized decision-making pillar. It needs to account for independence of autonomous structures, with cohesion nevertheless maintained, preserving the system's unit and identity. In many countries, apart from observance of the same regulatory frameworks, the independence of sub-systems and organizations in the health system is vast.

The internal differentiation of the health system gives room for the emergence and reproduction of several organizations, nevertheless sharing the same sense of identity of being operators in the same health system. This includes numerous healthcare service providers, as well as several organizations with system-wide overarching roles, concerned with observing, normative, oversight etc. across entities operating in the system.

The differentiation of service providers and non-service providers endows the system with sophisticated self-observation and self-organization competences, bringing it to a higher level of complexity. This internal differentiation of the system creates partial systems with specific roles. In this way, the system acquires capacity to orient its own reproduction without losing its central communication references and basic codification of operations related to service provision.

The partial system constituted by councils, associations, quality monitoring entities, accreditation, licensing organs, disciplinary regulators, etc. bring into health systems the mechanisms to guarantee compliance with basic normative codes. Such bodies oversee practices to ensure their legitimacy and correspondence to acceptable recognizable standards within the system. The influence of such bodies is felt inside each healthcare service delivery organization, as they assimilate standards and incorporate internal mechanisms of supervision and assessment of compliance by their respective professionals. The stability effect thus gained by the system is of enormous consequence. Every organization, by adopting the required standards and acknowledging the consequences of not doing so, is at the same time monitored by the other organizations, in mutual observation of their commitments to the same sets of rules binding everyone together. Without the autonomous adhesion and compliance of service providers to common standards, the task of the regulatory and normative sub-systems would be ineffective and irrelevant, and basically impossible.

The evolution of a health system, from underdeveloped configurations to high levels of complexity, can be traced by following how the sets of providers evolved together in their adoption of higher standards of care and regulatory compliance, simultaneously with the creation and capacity building of supervisory and regulatory bodies, performing their functions independently but still as components of the system (Foucault 2003).

The governance effects of such components cannot be understated. The proposition and approval of any legislation regulating aspect of health services provision, although established in the political system (not in the health system), are implemented by the health system itself. The health system maintains its control over the means of its own reproduction, or, in other words, its internal communications on adoption of regulations and practices. No other system has the legitimacy to do that for the health system.

Regulation implies observation and control. The governance pillar is meant to comprehend such internal self-regulatory dynamics of the system, but in fact the self-regulation systemic function goes beyond the exercise of governing the system by a ministry of health with its dissemination of norms, policies, guidelines, etc. supposed to orient all actors in the system. Several mechanisms of self-observation and self-regulation that are performed by the subsystems themselves do not correspond to the operations considered to be part of the governance pillar.

Yes, regulations establish standards of observation and related communications. However, a partial-system like a hospital deliberates continuously and autonomously on rules to be followed. That includes from setting up simple daily routines to major structural changes in line with legal or macro-policy determinations. Once a rule is set, further observations are required to check compliance and results. And additional cycles of communication are set in motion for monitoring, information processing and decision-making. The hospital itself takes care of all of that.

Therefore, the two functions – self-observation and self-regulation – are carried out in tandem, eliciting and orientating the self-reproduction of elements of the system. Obviously, small healthcare centres staffed with a nurse and midwife would have a small range of decisions to make at its discretion compared to a large and complex hospital. Nevertheless, if an element of the system has any degree of autonomy in organizing and setting up its routines, it will conduct self-observation and self-regulation in whatever way it can in order to reduce the complexities it faces. This is part of the distributed manner by which centrally enacted policies and rules are reprocessed, adjusted and followed according to the competences at the level of each component of the system.

Besides, there are many other arrangements that the components need to design and integrate into their functionality, which are not determined by any enacted rules at higher or central hierarchical or political levels. The exercise of autonomy may or may not be subject to supervisory and compliance monitoring, but the absence of such controls do not eliminate the capacity of the components to take initiatives and therefore self-observe and self-regulate. This can be rather a matter of survival of the components than of just complying with or corresponding to requirements of governance rules.

When staff in health facilities take under-the-table payments from patients, this may be against the explicit rules of the system, but could be essential for the continuity of services in adverse circumstances, for instance when salaries are too low or not regularly paid. The informal fees may guarantee the permanency of the professionals as well as the continuity of the services and perhaps the survival of the overall system.

Concluding remarks

Obviously, the notion of Six Pillars is a simplification of what is in fact observed in any health system. There is no question that the idea of pillars as bearers of the larger structures above them reflects the essential elements for the operations of the system: medicines, finances, human resources, information, etc. These are fundamental inputs for healthcare delivery. The metaphor of the pillar expresses this composition of essential elements sustaining the overall structure. But, at the same time, this symbolic representation does not facilitate awareness of the complexities it hides.

Yes, the notion of pillars is simple and useful. It calls planners' and researchers' attention to essential elements of a health system. However it leaves unanswered questions on how to reconcile the notion of pillars with the concept of system and its autonomous parts.

A few concluding remarks are pertinent. Health systems pillars are not conceptualized as units of the health system; they rather encompass structures and functions that independently operate and are spread out across many levels, among several organizations of the health system. While sets of indicators reflecting pillars' composition and dimensions (WHO 2010) give valuable aggregated pictures of relevant elements for country-level macro-planning, at less aggregated and more operational level, the organized component units of the system deal with elements of the pillars as their own resources, know-how and practices, not as macro-pillars sustaining the system.

A health organization, independently from the macro-aggregated attributes of the pillars of the overall system, deals with its resources not as elements of pillars but rather as components or its "production function", which needs to be optimized with little concern about what the macro-planning foresees.

An important conclusion to draw from this discussion is that the conceptualization of the Six Pillars, despite its contribution to macro planning of health systems, still lacks the actual systemic view crucial for conceiving initiatives to strengthen health systems.

Of course, better human resources, higher budgets, effective health information systems, comprehensive packages of medicines, and so on, improve the performance of the system and make it better able to deliver what is expected from it, i.e. more and better health services.

But this does not address health as a system. Those investments correspond to traditional managerial approaches, where the health system is seen as a large organization of service provision, expected to use inputs and control mechanisms, according to production functions, to generate outputs, in the same way as for any large enterprise. There is little systems insight in such approach, apart from the input–output and the interconnectedness of the parts as described in models of the very early stages of general systems science.

Chapter 1 – Niklas Luhmann's Social Systems Theory – Concepts

This chapter introduces the concepts of Luhmann's Social Systems Theory. Luhmann's books provide explanations of the central concepts of the theory; three of them present comprehensive definitions (Luhmann 1995, 2007, 2013). In the following paragraphs we use definitions taken from those three sources.

Luhmann provided definitions for a number of concepts that already existed; the concepts therefore acquired meanings they did not previously have. In this chapter the concepts are presented in simple terms in glossary format. In subsequent chapters, where the concepts are used in the discussions, richer and more detailed definitions are given.

To begin with, we need to consider that the overall architecture of the theory is based on the distinction of autopoietic and non-autopoietic systems. Among the autopoietic system we find three types of systems: the biological, the psychic and the social system. Luhmann's sociology is obviously concerned exclusively with social systems. The details come next.

System Luhmann says: "system is the difference between system and environment" (Luhmann 2013, p. 44). This definition gives us the key notion that the system–environment distinction is the fundament of the creation of a system. The systems appear and are therefore observable as a result of this distinction, by which the observer can assign the place of observation either inside the system or in the environment. In other words, this distinction is the key constitutive step of social systems – systems come to exist as distinct from environment. A social system does not appear without its environment; for instance, health systems are orientated towards diseases happening in its environment. Once a disease is detected, communications about it become part of the health system. A system can internally consider its constitutive distinction, making for itself an internal representation of the environment that concerns it. Within the environment, anything irrelevant for system's operations is not a matter of concern for the system. The system can also recognize the presence of other systems in the environment.

Autopoiesis Imported from the works of the biologists Humberto Maturana and Francisco Varela (1974) and applied by Luhmann to Social Systems, autopoiesis is understood as the driving basal orientation of social systems. It denotes the condition of existence of social systems, consisting in self-reproducing through the means they themselves produce. A social system either performs its autopoiesis or does not exist as a system; and no system can take care of the reproduction of any other system. Social systems are therefore orientated towards assuring the preservation of their self-reproduction, which implies preserving the consistency of generating capabilities of the means of reproduction. Autopoiesis is also a permanent drive, performed at each operation of the system, and no system can afford to "take a break" in that regard. Where there is a social system, autopoiesis is at work at all times.

Communication Communication is, so to speak, the "building block" of social systems. Luhmann uses the term communication with meanings distinct from the traditional transmission model of communication, where "Alter" sends a message that is then received by "Ego", thus completing the communication link. For Luhmann, in contrast, communication has three components: content (information), utterance and understanding. Utterance is the physical emission (sound vibration, visible printed characters, light signals, tactile braille, etc.), and content is the conveyed information (within a given shared semantic universe of significances). Understanding is the unit of content and utterance, and is what make possible the interlacing and exchange with the subsequent utterances and contents. Without such interlacing, which may consist for example in a request for clarification, we cannot say that communication has occurred. In this sense, understanding includes misunderstanding. In Luhmann's terms, social systems are made up of communications and nothing else; in other words, without communication there is no social system. Communication has attributes of recursive confirmation and self-validation, interlacing past, present and future communications, stabilizing meanings and the systems that rely on them. Furthermore, for Luhmann society is the totality of the communications taking place, and no communication takes place outside society.

Contingent and double contingency Contingent means something that could be different, i.e. in its current forms and attributes it is neither necessary nor impossible. All communications happen in a condition of double contingency, which means that on both sides Alter and Ego, while engaging in communication, know that they are performing their own selections over what is said, listened and replied to. The selections Ego makes can be different from Alter's and vice versa. The selections include the possibility of rejection of the communicated messages. All social systems have to live with the improbability of understanding, given the contingent selections, and also the open possibility of rejection.

Operational closure A key-structuring feature of a social system is the closure; a system can only deal with the information it internally produces. No information in the environment can be taken in directly by a system. What is observed in the environment becomes information once the perceptions are selected and internally processed. Operational closure correlates with autopoiesis in the sense that the selection and validation of observations and communications are prerogatives (and survival matters) of the system, and no other system can insert information inside another system; in the same way, a mind (a psychic system) cannot put a thought inside another mind (another psychic system). If that was possible, the boundaries of the two systems would collapse and the system/environment distinction would no longer be valid. Operational closure nevertheless allows for a system s capacity not only to observe itself but also to observe another.

Three types of social systems In his grand sociological theory, Luhmann differentiates three types of social systems: function systems, organizations and interactions. Each type is defined in terms of the specific ways they communicatively operate within their closure. *Function systems* are based on specific binary codes of communications (see next point); *organizations* are systems based on membership and decisions (a specific type of communication); *interactions* are short-lived systems constituted by face-to-face communications. A function system, like the health system, does not exclude anyone in the society as either user or provider can take part in it at some point. Differently, organizations select those it can identify and can identify themselves as members (employees for instance), and only members can take part in valid decision-making communications. Interactions are communication systems that develop where two or more people meet (face-to-face or virtually) and once the communication is over the system ceases. Obviously society members may take part in several social systems, sometimes simultaneously.

Binary codes   Binary codes are essential for identity building of *function systems*. We do not refer here to the other two types of systems as explained previously: *organization* and *interaction*. Each *function system* has its own specific binary code (legal/illegal, healthy/sick, government/opposition, art/not art, etc.). The binary codes mark and are fundamental to all communications as communications of the specific *function system*. No *function system* has the capability and legitimacy to use the code that belongs to another *function system*. The society does not recognize a communication stating that something is legal or illegal if such communication comes from any *function system* but the system of law. The words legal and illegal can be used in any circumstances but they will not carry the weight, legitimacy and consequences of, for instance, an adjudication of a court of law. Society members with professional attribution inside the health system would clearly distinguish the communications on health matters that are valid. *Function systems* are therefore based in simple binary codes that nevertheless can provide infinite possibilities of ramifications in increasing levels of complexity.

Structural coupling   Complementary to the concept of operational closure, structural coupling recognizes the possibility of systems observing each other, and by doing so achieve some level of coordination, nevertheless keeping their closure. In Luhmann's terms, systems organized under their respective constitutive closure do find ways to observe others and by doing so "irritate" or "are irritated by" the other, creating expectations and reacting to other systems without losing their distinctive separation from the environment and the other systems in it. *Structural coupling* is the term Luhmann uses to describe such operations; it allows for coordination between different social systems, like health and education, health and law, etc., as each system can observe the others, selecting what is relevant for each, and in the process operate in a coordinated manner as seen from the observer's point of view.

Social differentiation   In Luhmann's grand theory, the current stage of evolutionary transformation of societies' structures is characterized by the existence of several operationally closed and differentiated *function systems*. From previous stages of *segmented* and *stratified* societies, historical evolution has arrived at the advanced stage of social differentiation that started in the eighteenth century. Differentiated *function systems* (law, politics, economics, health, religion, art, media, etc.) create addresses whereby inclusion of individuals is open to all society members, preserving the possibility for anyone to be concurrently included to varying degrees in several function systems. Differentiated function systems strive to keep their characteristics and specificities with socially precisely recognizable boundaries between them, mainly based on their binary codes and communications. At the *segmented* society stage, individuals were assigned to social structures by their place of birth or life. *Stratified* societies were more complex and individuals were assigned to a stratus the society created (such as castes, social classes, artisanal groups, etc.). In the modern society, differentiated in *function systems*, no function system has the central role and preponderates over the others; even the political functional system is one functional system among the others.

Distinctions and observations An important turn in the development of Social System Theory is Luhmann's incorporation of the works of the mathematician George Spencer-Brown. In the *Laws of Form*, Spencer-Brown (2015) asserts the inseparability of observations and distinctions. To make observations, one needs to draw distinctions. Distinctions are forms with two sides: the marked and the unmarked. A distinction is thus a unit of difference. Observations are made according to the adopted distinctions. To carry out an observation, the observer takes the marked side, which is of interest – for instance, disease instead of health – and leaves the rest out, on the unmarked side. These are essential selection processes by which systems can become self-referential, self-observing and self-organizing (see these definitions later). Furthermore, all observation has blind spots[1]; the blind spot is often the deployed distinction itself. A distinction can also be observed, but that requires another distinction assigning the distinction to be observed to the marked side.

Second-order observation Another important reference in the development of Luhmann's theory is the works of Foerster (2014), who conceptualized the cybernetic qualitative step by which an observing system can observe observers and, respectively, the distinctions they use and the observations they make. This includes self-observation. All social systems perform first- and second-order observations.

---

1   Observers need to distinguish themselves from what they observe, in doing so, to carry out the observation, they stay in the "blind spot".

Coding and programming Coding is the way of orientating communication. Binary codes offer the two sides of the distinctions the communication refers to, while always electing one side. Programmes guide the selection of themes and semantics, supporting communication connectivity within the chosen side of the binary distinction.

Complexity Complexity is a feature of observation, not a reality in itself. It denotes that both a system and its environment have elements and relations between elements that surpass the system's observation capacity. A system has to reduce complexity, by making selections and focusing on relevant internal and/or external elements, excluding the rest from consideration. Complexity therefore refers to the unavoidable limits in the capacity of making observations. Contingency is intrinsic to complexity, because while reducing complexity a system has to make selections, which by their turn could be different, i.e. are contingent. The environment is more complex than the systems.

Having briefly described these central concepts, there is moreover a relevant set of specific concepts. Luhmann's studies in the field of management science have attracted attention among those interested in organizations as social systems. Health systems have many organizations and therefore it is relevant to understand how this type of system (organization) operates. The conceptual understanding of organizations includes the following:

Decision Decision is a particular type of communication crucial for the existence of organizations. Without decision there is no organization. All matters of concern for an organization as social system are objects of decisions. A decision communicates the side of the distinctions the subsequent communications should be connected to, therefore orientating and creating the premises for the decisions to be taken next.

Membership The differentiation between who belongs (members) and who does not belong to an organization is of vital importance for any organization. All organizations are based on decisions and membership, and only members take legitimate decisions, or, in other words, only decisions taken by members are recognized as valid and relevant for the organization.

Uncertainty absorption A decision already made does not have to communicate the uncertainties that surrounded it before it was taken, which include the ambiguities or doubts in relation to the evidence and inferences guiding the decision. A communicated decision does not communicate that it is also contingent, i.e. the possibility that the decision could be different. Once adopted, a decision thus absorbs uncertainties, which are then excluded from further consideration. The absorption of uncertainties achieved by decisions is therefore crucial for the management of any organization.

Decision premises Decision premises is a functional characteristic of decisions that make former decisions the justifications for subsequent ones, thus becoming the basis of organizations' life. Decision premises help to solve the paradoxical nature of any decision; the paradox of undecided decisions which derives from the fact that if an option is obviously better than all the others, there is no decision to be made; conversely, if all options are equally good, a decision cannot be made. So, decision premises attract and justify the choice in terms of the decisions previously made. Luhmann identified three types of decision premises: programmes (with stabilized sets of prescriptions and expectations), personnel (with stabilized definitions of members' roles) and communication channels (also understood as organizational culture, setting courses for routine formal and informal communication flows). Decisions based on decision premises have the advantage of not having to exhaustively demonstrate the reasons for taking them.

There are a number of additional important concepts with rather complex formulations. They are briefly mentioned and explained as advanced topics in the Annex.

Having presented the central concepts of the Social System Theory, the next section discusses the differences between Luhmann's formulations and the more traditional views that Luhmann's theory does not incorporate. Three topics are discussed: 1) the *input–output model*; 2) the notion of a *system as bigger than the sum of its parts*; and 3) the concept of the *adaptive system* and its evolution.

These topics are not required for understanding Luhmann's theory and therefore readers, particularly those following health systems thinking approaches, may want to be aware of the reasons behind Luhmann's theoretical decisions, and their implications. Those who are only familiar with those commonly held views about systems are particularly encouraged to read the section, and familiarize themselves with Luhmann's explanations for not including these views in his conceptual architecture. The discussion is rich and instructive, and builds on a number of the concepts presented in the first section of this chapter.

1. The input–output model

"The systems thinking approach goes beyond this 'input-blackbox-output' paradigm to one that considers inputs, outputs, initial, intermediate and eventual outcomes, and feedback, processes, flows, control and contexts" (WHO 2009, p. 34). In common with this understanding, Luhmann's theory moves away from the input–processing–output model predominant in the 1950s and earlier.

In his theory, however, inputs are not taken in, processed and the resultant "products" sent to the environment as outputs. Inputs are creations of the system. The system does not take in what it observes in the environment; it interprets and translates what is observed into meaningful information, consistent with the meanings the system has at its disposal and works with.

Luhmann says that there is no information as such in the environment. Information does not penetrate the system; it is instead generated inside the system. Surely, though, a system relies on the sources of energy and materials in the environment. This, however, is a basic distinction that needs to be considered, separating the physical world and the world of communications and meanings.

For any biological organism, energy and materials do enter the body, and the waste is subsequently thrown out. The same does not happen with information. As said earlier, information does not enter; it is elaborated inside the system. A system may make available the results of its information processing to other systems; but it can neither insert the information into the other system nor enforce it, if the other system does not observe it or consider the information relevant.

Luhmann therefore uses the words input and output with very specific connotations; inputs and outputs are recognized as such inside the system, in the way it internally and communicatively processes the information it generates itself. These points have implications for the theoretical conceptualization of the closedness and openness of systems.

A number of questions therefore become pertinent. For instance: how open can a system be and still preserve its boundaries and identities? How close can a system be and still acquire energy, and make observations for its information processes without running the risk of being annihilated by the environment?

The theory offers the following considerations. Systems can only translate what they observe in the environment into information because they are operationally closed. If information could penetrate the system, it would be the same as someone inserting their own thoughts inside someone else's mind, as mentioned previously. The distinction between the two minds would collapse and both minds consequently would have the same fate. Although they cannot take information from the environment, the systems can take energy and materials from it; they are therefore both open and closed.

Thus understood, operational closure, deriving from the basic system/environment distinction, is the very condition for the system to process observations and elaborate information. As the environment is incomparably more complex than the system, the system does not have what is conceptually denominated as "requisite variety" (Luhmann 2013, p. 121) by which it could establish complete representation inside the system, relating one to one all the elements in the environment. Therefore, the system needs to make selections of what it is going to process and observe in the environment. This reduces environmental complexities as far as the system is concerned, without affecting the environment, which remains as complex as before.

If these notions are accepted, it is understandable that the system would be destroyed by the overwhelming volume of information the environment could potentially generate. If information as such were coming from the environment and entering the system, the system would not be able to distinguish what belonged to it as opposed to the environment. Information generation therefore is a process in which systems are actively engaged as a matter of autopoietic survival.

Still in relation to the input–output model, the notion of "non-trivial systems" (Foerster 2014) is relevant to consider. A non-trivial system may process and generate diverse types of outputs with the same observation it makes in its environment. This system can observe itself, and therefore it can reflect on its own processes and results, and introduce changes, which as a result may render the generated outputs unpredictable for an external observer.

Compared to the simple rather outdated input–process–output model, these models of self-referred systems dynamics grant a conceptual architecture with better tools to approach the complexities of social systems such as the health system. Translating these understandings into observations of health systems' operations we can see as follows.

A case of a suspected disease remains an unknown event in the environment among all sorts of events taking place in it. Once it is detected by a health professional, which then communicates about it inside the health system, the suspected disease becomes a point of reference so that subsequent communications can take place in the system. Before it was detected, it was not information waiting to be disclosed; it was just an unknown.

Disease detection is carried out by procedures of observations whereby health professionals deploy the distinctions they were trained to use. The health professionals write the reports or communicate orally what they observe. From that moment on, the event "unknown disease" acquires the form of "symptoms and suspected diagnostic", which can be recognized, read, checked, registered, etc., becoming in the process a communicated reality within the system.

The information can then be retrieved, coded, double-checked, criticized, complemented, and so on, according to the programmes the system communicatively deploys. The former "unknown" therefore acquires "life", so to speak, as a disease inside the system. Effectively, by becoming communicatively inserted in the system, the disease actually becomes part of the system as a recognizable event/object.

The self-reference (including self-observation and self-organization) functionality of the system endows it with the capacity to adjust its observational capacities, refine its interpretation and service delivery capabilities, and proceed with the autopoietic reproduction of these abilities. All that will be in correspondence with the (internal and external) level of complexity the system can handle.

The reproduction of the system therefore can only be self-reproduction, because only the system understands and can use the communications that are its prerogatives. The input–processing–output model does not give a proper account of these highly relevant systemic functions.

2. The system is bigger than the sum of its parts

Systems are more than the sum of their parts is perhaps the most commonly held view about systems. At first glance, it seems there is nothing wrong with that, as the statement calls attention to functions emerging out of a collection of elements, which individually and separately do not show those specific functionalities.

However, this concept of the whole and parts cannot easily accommodate the notion that social systems are made of communications. While the idea of parts physically and functionally distinct and the whole that encompasses them is easily perceived in systems that have precise concrete existence, such as ecological systems, nervous systems, urban transport systems and so on, it is less evident when comes to intangible realities, such as social systems based on communications. The whole and parts concept does not seem to give a good account of the set-up of the system.

The argumentation that follows looks at the *whole/parts* from the Social Systems Theory perspective, which includes discussions on the validity of the scheme considering that: 2.1) systems are made of communications; 2.2) communications cannot be summed up like "bricks"; 2.3) communications interlace each other making stable 'meaning pools";[2] 2.4) communications not only make the system but also reproduce it; 2.5) communications make the internal differentiations and sub-systems; 2.6) communications differentiate a system from other systems in its environment; and, finally, 2.7) the *whole/parts* scheme is analysed as a potential observation device deployed by a system for self-reference and self-organization.

2.1 Systems as communications

Questions concerning a system's parts and whole acquire new difficulties when we consider that systems are made of communications, as proposed by the Social Systems Theory. How can parts of a system add up to a whole if they are identified as communications?

A nervous system can be dissected and its parts isolated even in organisms still alive. If a part is severed, the reaction at the level of the whole system can be monitored. The parts can be identified and counted; the connections between them can be cut or preserved. Some parts may play a more important role than others in terms of the overall emergent functionality of the system.

However, if we take communications as the parts of the system, a piece of isolated communication no longer constitutes part of the system, because what makes a communication part of the system is the fact that it is connected to other communications belonging to the system; the connectivity is crucial.

Communications are events connected to other communicative events. If a nurse observes that the temperature of the patient is rising and does not communicate that to the other nurses and doctors, the communication event that does not happen has not become part of the system.

But the system does not have an inventory of communications already established, representing the aggregation of all parts of the system. Commu-

---

2   These terms, "bricks" and "meaning pools", do not come from Luhmann.

nications cannot be dissected and counted. The virtual inventory of communications, if we may keep this expression, is being built as communications happen, as opposed to the stable list of components of a system with discrete countable identifiable parts that can be regularly inventoried.

The observation the nurse had made may never be incorporated into the universe of events constituting the health system. Similarly, a communication may happen and remain isolated, as for instance a note in the patient's dossier that was never considered and ended up forgotten in the archive (or database) of the hospital among hundreds of thousands of other records. In spite of communications that may not happen or have been forgotten, the system carries on its autopoiesis with all the other communications taking place. No single communication has the crucial role for the existence of a social system, as is the case in certain systems with core function such as the nervous system.

Unlike a system with a countable limited number of components, a system made of communication has an unlimited number of components and cannot correspond to any prescription of amounts of communications that need to take place and the time for that. In communication-based systems, the parts cannot be assembled together in a predefined permanent, stable combination, although routine communications may occur regularly. New communication parts will always be required.

These explanations should give a clear understanding of the specificities of social systems. Although themes and topics (such as those in the universe of specific medical specialties) create sets of communications related to each other and recurrently claiming continuity and consistency, the field of communication has to remain open because of both the nature of communication as events in time and the limitlessness resulting from the complexity of human health. Some additional considerations are still pertinent in relation to communication and the parts/whole scheme.

It must be clear now that a communication-based system is not composed of the elements communicating with each other inside it. It is not meaningful to count the communicating elements as if they were the individual parts of the system. We may see communication as emerging (or otherwise not existing) and also comprising a network-like web of recurrent and forward-moving connected communicative events, reproducing themselves, in potentially infinite forms, in the system being built by them. Communication emerges from communications, not from the material base where it happens.

In view of that, the incongruity of comparing the constitution of a whole with the sum of its parts becomes clear. With some irony, scholars who studied Luhmann's work (King and Thornhill- 2003, p. 10) say: "the whole is less than the sum of its parts". This may be understood from the perspective that at any given moment, only a limited number of communications actualizing the system is in fact occurring, compared to the countless repertoire of possible communications and the incalculable numbers of previous communications of the same system.

The point to be retained in this discussion is that the system is comprised of the communications that are making it, and communications are continuously linking past communications with current and future ones. Only communications can make a system perform its communicative functions. In Luhmann's words "only communication can communicate" (Luhmann 2002). In the case of health systems, this means communicating and reproducing the healthy/sick binary code and the programmes sustained by it over the course of communicatively realized diagnostics and treatments.

Furthermore, the whole of the system cannot be equated to the addition of communications that have already taken place. Past communications only contribute to building the system if they are currently linked to actual on-going communications; otherwise they are irrelevant. The system's whole would thus be an artificial abstraction of the entire set of communications taking place in each given moment. Such abstraction is of no relevance.

2.2 Building blocks metaphor

Not all individuals identifiable as operating within the system are actually engaged in communications at all times. While the majority may remain "silent" and a small minority actually communicates at any given time, this does not mean that the system becomes smaller or bigger because there are fewer or more silent individuals.

The metaphor of "building block" implies the wrong impression of quantifiable accumulative unitary bricks. Communication cannot simply be reduced to countable discrete units of exchanges between individuals. Communications are more complex than that; as already mentioned, they imply connectivity with other communications.

It does not make sense either to compare parts of the system without communications, and parts of the system with communications, because there is only the system where communications occurs (whatever the time required). The parts of a communication-based social system are the communications taking place, not the members that could possibly communicate with each other.

The system does not include the communications that did not occur, even if they remained potential and plausible. Possible communications are not retrievable as recorded memory of the system and cannot interlace new communications. Consequently, if one still wants to use the simplistic "building block" metaphor, one needs to focus on the actual communications happening inside the system at any given time.

Of course communications vanish as soon as they happen, but this does not mean that systems disappear with them. Elements remain latent whether communications are taking place or not. For instance, the semantics, codes, grammars, syntaxes, symbols, semiotics, associated meanings, memories, etc. deployed during communications are kept as reservoirs of shapers of an infinite number of possible communications. The operators inside the system draw from those common stable memory pools the rules and signifiers needed to compose their messages, enabling them to be understood by the recipient of the messages, who uses the same pools for communicative purposes. Individuals' insertion in a system is preceded and maintained through continuous learning of those pools, allowing them to engage in meaningful communications inside the system. Memory plays a crucial role in this.

However, anything in those reservoirs that is not used becomes irrelevant as constitutive of the system. In the same way, information a health worker does not communicate back to the system's counterparts cannot be considered part of the system. The reservoirs are not accumulation of "building blocks"; the system thus should not be confused with those reservoirs and potential communications. A social system made up of communication does not have to make exhaustive uninterrupted use of all communications possibilities that can be produced with what is available in the pools. If that were the case, the system would be destroyed instantaneously. For that matter, the system makes selections. Any communication implies selections from both sides (sender and receiver), and cannot be otherwise. Selections are an inextricable part of communications, and therefore also constitutive operations of the system.

2.3 Interlacing communications

As explained in the first section of this chapter, communications are comprised of utterance, content (information) and understanding (including misunderstanding).³ They interlace with components of other communications, becoming part of a system. In isolation, an utterance or content is not integrated into a system. Communications always have the possibility of interlacing other communications on the accepting (yes) or the rejection (no) side, and through the content and/or the utterances. The recipient may emphasize either of these components while participating in communication.

By interlacing with others, a communication becomes part of meaningful sets of communications. The interlacing is thus fundamental to keep the system alive, and involves connectivity through both utterances and content. What we are trying to say here is that the importance of interlacing makes the cut-off of communication in discrete pieces irrelevant. It is rather artificial to cut a communication with the purpose of counting the numbers when the very fact of being meaningfully interlaced is the crucial aspect of communication.

2.4 Autopoiesis

Taking autopoiesis of systems into consideration, obviously a system does not carry out its self-reproduction without the concurrence of its parts. Clearly, when we speak about parts here we are talking about communications, nothing else. So, there would not be autopoiesis if the system did not reproduce the distinctive communications that characterize the system.

The communications are thus making the system, and at the same time realizing its autopoiesis. The communications thus reproduce previous communications and open connections for the subsequent ones. In this way, standards and semantics are meaningfully preserved and reproduced, assuring the continuity of the communicative operations of the system. Social systems reproduction is achieved through reproduction of its communications communications reproduce communications, we may say.

2.5 Internal differentiation

Let's consider now that communication can become specialized and differentiated inside a system. There may be sets of related communications, using specific semantics and selections, which may become characteristic of some

---

3   Luhmann says "understanding" is the unit of the distinction between "utterance" and "content".

identifiable sections, programmes or sub-systems of the encompassing system. These sub-systems become constitutive parts of the system, making it more complex.

A way of approaching the system/sub-systems distinction may use the concepts of integration and differentiation. Differentiation is one of the central concepts of Luhmann's theory; it refers to both the differentiation of systems in the same environment, and the internal differentiation of components inside a system. Integration, on the other hand, is not a key concept in the theory and Luhmann summarizes it as reduction of degrees of freedom of any system, while entering structural coupling with other systems.

Differentiation across systems is an outcome of the autopoiesis processes each system undertakes, while preserving their operational closure. By making their individual reproductive selections, any system becomes increasingly different from the others also performing their own autopoiesis in the same environment.

Internal differentiation, on the other hand, has to be understood as part of the individual dynamic process of autopoiesis itself. The system creates internal divisions in its processes of reproducing itself.[4] Internal differentiation increases a system's complexity and consequently the complexity the system can address in its environment.

A system may have internal parts involved in the processes of communicating the core business of the system (for instance, diagnostics and treatments in the health system). But it may also create parts specialized in self-observation of the system (monitoring and evaluation of health programmes for instance). The system may also have sections specialized in observing the environment (epidemiological surveillance and infectious diseases controls), and sections fulfilling normative roles, assessing if internal communications and actions correspond to the patterns and standards the system adopts (professional councils and ethical boards, for example).

Internal differentiation does not imply the creation of a distinct part with the attribution to rule the entire system on all matters. Some rules may be enacted, but only become effective when the parts incorporate them. The parts themselves perform coordinated acts to a large extent independently from central observation and control. Just think about how patients' referral systems may operate across health facilities, with facilities communicating

---

4 Reproducing internally the system/environment distinction.

with each other, sending and receiving patients without resorting to any centralized mechanism of authorization or subordination.

What should be retained from this discussion is that a system surely allows for the development of differentiated forms of communications between its components. But, in short, it is not relevant whether internal differentiation makes the whole bigger than the sum of its parts or otherwise. What matters is that it makes the whole internally diverse and better able to deal with the complexities of the environment, while preserving its unity and maintaining the distinctive character of the internal communications.

2.6 System-environment distinction

Perhaps crucial for understanding how Social Systems Theory deals with the parts/whole scheme is the notion that the system is, in Luhmann's words, "the difference between system and environment" (Luhmann 2013, p. 44). A system exists from the moment it becomes distinct from its environment. As a consequence, the maintenance of the system implies the maintenance of its differentiation vis-à-vis its environment.

The reproduction of a social system is the repetition of its system/environment difference and respective limits inside the system in all new sub-systems created, which individually repeat the original distinction, whatever specific additional functionalities the sub-systems may acquire. This is an advanced complex topic we can deal with later.

But, in this sense, a system is found where there is a system/environment distinction, not where there are parts comprising wholes. Social Systems Theory thus replaces the paradigm of the whole and parts difference with the difference between system and environment.

Parts can be arbitrarily aggregated without constituting a unit with a singular self-reference, clear delimitation in relation to the environment and without a cohesive process of self-reproduction and self-preservation. Think of a crowd in a busy train station – the collection of individual-parts does not make that a system.

To further illustrate this conception consider, for instance, a large bazaar with hundreds of independent stalls selling thousands of different products to thousands of buyers on a daily basis. If we take the whole and parts paradigm, we can say that there is a system here: the bazaar is the system and the shops its parts.

However, if we look at the collection of shops, consumers and products thus described and try to understand it from the point of view of the system/environment distinction we reach a different conclusion. We would have difficulty finding the operations the bazaar performs that sets the boundaries between it and what can be identified as its environment. If we exclude the managerial services of the bazaar, in charge of keeping the structures in working condition and renting out the stalls, there are no other overarching functions bringing a sense of unit.

As we see when we visit a bazaar, there is space for tens of thousands of daily buying/selling transactions. The administration of the bazaar can be identified as an organization (a type of social system). The stalls are not part of that organization. They act independently, renting the space and conducting their buying and selling operations as autonomous entities. Some coordination for determination of prices and selection of products may or may not happen; it will largely depend on the individual decisions of the stalls and administrators. However, they do react to what they observe taking place around them.

In this sense, the bazaar would rather be the environment where customers appear, observe products and prices and are observed by the stalls. Negotiations may happen and may evolve into a final selling and buying transaction. An analogy can be made, comparing customers in the environment of the bazaar and patients coming from the neighbourhood to get treatment in a primary healthcare centre. The communications involved in selling and buying in an economic system are functional equivalents to the communication operations involved in treating and receiving treatment in a health system. In both cases the system/environment distinction is more relevant in analytical terms than the parts/whole distinction, because the system configures itself vis-à-vis and in contrast with its environment.

In radical contrast with the whole and parts paradigm, the analysis from the point of the Social Systems Theory would conclude that the bazaar is in fact the environment instead of a system. Furthermore, we can also say that the bazaar does not perform autopoiesis; the environment does not do self-reproduction. Autopoiesis is a specific attribute of the systems.

2.7 Parts, wholes and observation

A final consideration on the parts and wholes topic suggests that the scheme can be understood as an observation strategy. In this sense, there is no ontological or technical prescription setting the sizes and limits of the parts to be considered. The questions about how big/small a part should be to be considered as a part do not have a definitive answer. The observer draws the distinctions, makes the definitions and proceeds to observe, describe and count the parts, according to his/her decisions, which are all contingent (i.e. could be different).

In object-orientated ontology, Graham Harman (2018) says an object can be approached and described by cutting it into its component parts or by relating it to other objects. These approaches can also be employed jointly. The limit is that the object can never be apprehended in itself. Parts and wholes are thus deployed observational techniques. The question whether the whole is more than the sum of its parts depends on the understanding of the attributes being observed and their relevance or irrelevance as attributes of the parts or of the whole. So, the results of cutting into parts are contingent, and do not reveal the essential nature of the object.

We think these conclusions sit comfortably with the conclusions Social Systems Theory suggests to us. If the parts of the object system are communications, they cannot meaningfully be summed up to the totality of a single whole that is graspable as the defined object within which all its parts are accommodated. The system object would not be apprehended in itself.

Furthermore, for observation purposes, the notion of parts implies the assumption that they are homogeneous or at least have common uniform qualities that all parts show in some strictly comparable manner. But, as Luhmann (1995, p. 7) says, "there were hardly any theoretically proven criteria for homogeneity".

Hospitals, public health programmes, professional bodies, etc. can be considered as sub-systems of a health system. For that, they may only have the fact of being orientated towards and mobilized by the communication concerning healthy/sick binary code in one of its multiple presentations and focus. In other words, the fact that these sub-systems are included in the universe of communications recognized as exclusively belonging to the health system attests to their insertion in the overall health system.

Therefore, sub-systems are part of the health system as legitimate makers of health communications, regardless of the size or quantity of each sub-system's communications. The semantic order the sub-system is inserted into does not require specific homogeneity of their messages, or specific sizes of their sentences, or specific effects of their utterances, or specific complexity of the information conveyed, or specific quantity of exchanges, or comparative relevance or frequency in relation to communications of other sub-systems.

Any measurement of communications in such ways would be meaningless. The semantic order, by means of autopoietic self-reference and self-reproduction, attests the validity of the communications as part of the system.

For its self-reproduction, the system may see advantages in adopting the parts/whole observation scheme, when the technique may facilitate the system's internal communication about itself. In this process, semantic spaces are created, configuring sub-systems, as might be the case for example in the creation of communications specific to medical specialities. The self-reference thus achieved and maintained contributes to the autopoiesis of the system. The question whether the whole is or isn't bigger than the sum of its parts remains irrelevant from the system's self-reproduction and self-reference perspective. In its self-reflection, a system will look for ways of reducing its own complexities; the more complex a system becomes, the less it will try to create a copy of itself that reflects all its complexities, it will therefore settle with self-descriptions that summarize the main features the system is selectively electing as its priorities, vis-à-vis the environment from which it distinguishes itself. In conclusion, the parts/whole scheme should be employed according to internal self-observation aims, if this deployment is to have some advantage.

3. The notion of adaptive systems

Health systems are "complex adaptive systems" (Olivier, J. et al. 2017, p. 21). Throughout the health systems thinking literature one finds references as such to health systems as complex adaptive systems (CAS). This is a potentially controversial topic, if one considers what the Social Systems Theory says about the concept of adaptation.

If adaptation only means learning and incorporating new information into its communications, social systems are indeed adaptive; this is partially consistent with the Social Systems Theory. Adaptation in this case refers exclusively to internal changes in the system, without necessarily linking it with better chances of survival in a given environment. Learning is operationally achieved by the necessary connections between past, current and future communications, establishing new and more complex memories and repertoires of themes, which the system uses for processing information.

Nevertheless, if adaptive refers to adaptation to an external environment (however it may be defined), it is necessary to consider that the theory highlights the system's environment as a construction of the system itself; the system selects in the environment the elements it observes and considers relevant for its autopoiesis, ignoring the rest. In the process, the system is aligned with the environment itself is recurrently confirming and constructing. The understanding of the founding role of the system/environment distinction in the theory is therefore crucial to approaching the adaptation issue.

The following example may help this discussion. Take a hospital as a system (an organization system in line with the theory), and its emergency ward overwhelmed by the number of cases arriving at its door. The hospital may decide to set up a triage procedure, by which cases are sent through to one of the following four options: immediate care; referral to more complex centres; stay and wait; or send home. Some patients may voluntarily select themselves out and go to another hospital or home. This may be the case on a particularly busy Saturday night but might also be a trend observed over a number of months. With the triage, the hospital is selecting what it is observing in the environment (its doorstep).

What an external observer may see as system adaptation to a higher demand (the triage), an internal one sees it as a selection operation. For the hospital, it is not of primary relevance whether the procedure represents an adaptation to the environment or not. The procedure is a solution to the pressure the hospital-system is internally detecting; the hospital needs to safeguard its internal processes and communications against possible collapse. The hospital is primarily concerned with the integrity of its communication, its autopoiesis. Intervention in the environment beyond its doorstep is not its concern. The environment at large may carry on producing more and more cases (or not); the hospital is neither more nor less adapted to the case production capacity and its determinants in the environment. It is only carrying on its operations within the limits it recognizes as important for its operations; it is adjusting internal communicative operations, not aiming at achieving better adaptation to the environment. As an organizational system, the hospital is selecting from its environment the elements that it considers of interest and finds itself capable of handling. The crucial point is that internal adjustments do not necessarily represent adaptation to the environment.

The hospital could have continued its internal routines without the triage it has set up, maintaining ad hoc spontaneous triage as before. If the new procedure is considered an adaptation, it was an "adaptation to itself", learning and incorporating new elements, as noted at the beginning. The adjustments were intended to achieve better coordination, releasing tensions and stresses among the staff, and pressures on hospital resources. If any adaptation is happening, it is to the internal environment of the hospital. It can still be considered that these changes could be conceived and incorporated anyway, independently from the pressures of the external environment. The hospital could set up a triage for the advantages in handling the arriving cases and for preparedness, in case it expected to face a possible surge in demand in the near future.

In more theoretical terms, in *La Sociedad de la Sociedad*, Luhmann (2007a) speaks of an excess of possibilities the systems internally develop and try, which are not related, conductive or justified by the necessity of adaptation to the environment. The independence of the systems from the environment, allowing freedom for internal communications, endows systems with the capability to develop new distinctions, new forms for new observations, new ways of communicating and so on. This wealth of possibilities and subsequent adoption of changes leads to differentiations inside and among the systems, which do not necessarily rely on some sort of "natural selection" to survive and reproduce. The emergence of the peacock tail could not be explained if all a system could do (biological ones included) was to strictly adapt to its environment.

Luhmann (1995) also says no system has the "requisite variety" to internally represent the environment in all its complexities and control the "natural selection" adaptation. He says: "The system can only compensate the lack of knowledge of its environment with intern excess of possibilities, to say, can compensate the lack of determination in the environment with its own lack of determination". (p. 182).

He continues by explaining that the capacity of the system to draw its distinctions and use them to make observations in the environment (and itself) is a function that does not have any correlate in the environment. Distinctions are not imposed by the environment and do not exist as such in it. The capacity to independently draw distinctions endows the system with the possibility to create an excess of possible internal elements and configurations that it can adopt regardless of what the environment has.

Furthermore, where the system decides to closely couple with elements of the environment (other systems, for instance, as the health system couples with the political, economic, legal, etc. systems), it does so with its operational closure and autopoietic reproduction, where it sees the advantages of doing so. In other words, it selects the way it couples with other systems according to the calculations and information processing it is capable of.

On the other side, the overarching, all-encompassing environment is supportive (i.e. not strictly selective) of many possible forms the systems living in it autopoietically incorporates in themselves. The environment tolerates, so to speak, large variation of new individual and collective forms, no matter whether they are "fine-tuned" or not to the environment.

To be sure, selection may happen in the environment, but the environment does not perform autopoiesis. As the system can produce an excess of forms for its autopoiesis (not only the strictly determined ones), the environment has excess potentialities and expanded unused capabilities to absorb ever-increasing diversity of autopoietic systems with unknown limitations. As already said, the environment is not governed by autopoietic drive, so it does not "intentionally" make selections.

In conclusion, adaptation is a concept that does not grant the system privileged chances to perform its autopoiesis. A system cannot increase or decrease its autopoiesis or its chances to perform that. A system that stops its autopoiesis also stops its adaptation because it is already dead. In its autopoietic drive, a system is doing more than what the adaptation expects; it is varying its processes of reproduction and creation of the means to reproduce itself.

What tells a system whether the tested and adopted new operations and respective means of doing so should be maintained or not, is not the adaptation but rather the way the system recognizes it as feasible to be repeated and maintained, given, first of all, its internal communicative capabilities to do so. If adaptation to the environment is achieved – meaning, if the system's new ways of successfully reproducing itself do not meet strong negative reactions in the environment – this might be an additional argument for keeping going and inventing new forms.

It is something well established in biological sciences that although adaptation to the environment assures good chances of survival, it does not explain the huge variations of forms created, where surely some of them are in fact costly and represent a sub-optimal adaptation strategy; members of some species would have better chances of survival without some of the characteristics they have acquired, although the specie as a whole carries on faring well.

Having said that, a few additional reflections are necessary. The word "adaptive" has strong denotation associated with Darwinism and natural selection. It expresses the idea of "adaptation" of species (and more recently of psychological and social systems) to their environment. It is hard to use the word without such connotations. Adaptation is therefore understood as the driving process by which a system becomes better able to live in a given environment and by doing so becomes more resilient. The system–environment relation in such a notion is of determination, whereby the environment has the causal factors, which the system has to recognize and adjust accordingly.

Luhmann's Social Systems Theory departs from such notions in correspondence with his conceptualization of operationally closed systems built by communications. As already said, if there is adaptation, and Luhmann would not dismiss this possibility, he would qualify it as adaptation to an environment that the system represents internally, meaning "adaptation" to the represented environment with the selected features seen as relevant by the system, and not the environment itself in all its complexities.

Furthermore, not all transformation a system goes through is necessarily intended to make it better adapted to its environment. The autopoiesis of the system, by which the system reproduces itself through its own means, may generate internal structures of communication that are understood by the system as relevant in themselves for the systemic operations it keeps running.

For instance, when a health system hit by an epidemic elaborates and puts in place new structures and routines, it is adjusting itself to the internal tensions and pressures it observes in consequence of the increased number of cases of the disease. Is this system becoming better adapted to its environment? It is possible to say yes, because the pressure is coming from the environment and the system is trying to respond to it. However, whatever the system internally does cannot be summarily described as adaptation to the environment. Through its operational units the system is adjusting functionalities as is feasible within the units' capabilities and resources, and their competences to self-observe and select what needs to be changed (increased, or stopped, or reduced, or started anew, etc.). Each unit, as distinct organization systems (hospitals, clinical facilities, etc.), redesigns part of its internal functions according to its self-observation and self-organization capabilities. In that, each unit offer limited responses, taking into account and seeking coherence with all the other operations the unit has to keep running. It has, so to speak, the keys to the control room and the codes that can operate any transformation intended to offer better responses to the new pressures from the environment, as well as to better preserve the existing functionalities of the system, considering its regular routines, protecting existing functions from the new interferences.

The prerogatives and the priorities for keeping the system running and performing its autopoiesis overrule the circumstantial pressures coming from the environment. If not for that, the environment could destroy the system; the system must keep its selective capabilities – the ones it has acquired over the years, even if they are not optimal in face of changes in the environment.

Furthermore, if the current complexities of the system represent successful self-organization the system has adopted throughout its history, that does not mean the system could not be different today, and that the decisions previously taken couldn't have been different. Contingency is the concept that Luhmann often brings into these discussions. The decisions are contingent, meaning they could be different or even the opposite – a certain decision is neither necessary nor could it not be different. In this sense, if there is adaptation, it did not follow any directionality imposed by the environment. The system selected its new operations and the selection process is contingent, i.e. we repeat, it could be different.

This changes significantly our understanding of adaptation – not as deterministic but as a field of possibilities with some having a lower probability of being selected but nevertheless being chosen and implemented, leading to a future state of the system that is perfectly functional even if circumstantially less cost-effective.[5]

Understanding adaptation to the environment as a major driver of a system misses the point of the high contingency of the decisions a system can make and their subsequent success. "Adaptive" is therefore an adjective that can be easily used in reference to health systems but, first, it is not an object of clear scrutiny and specification, and second, even worse, it obstructs the sight of health systems' huge diversity, internal complexities and the contingencies of their decisions.

---

5   A large hospital complex may decide to install high-tech new equipment that can hardly bring investment returns, but nevertheless puts the hospital in the forefront of the advancing technologies that eventually will become routine; the hospital will then have gathered the necessary experience.

Chapter 2 – General application of the theory[1]

This chapter presents our attempts to describe the health system using the conceptual apparatus offered by Social System Theory. The discussion unfolds in three sections:

1. The first question to be addressed is whether health systems can be considered a *function system* according to Luhmann's conceptual architecture. In one of his few articles on health, Luhmann (2016)[2] agrees that health is indeed a *function system*; he speaks of "medical system" or a "system for treatment of the sick". This section discusses the basis for the categorization: the existence of binary code (healthy/sick), the autopoiesis, the operational closure, the social differentiation, the specific programmes, the coupling with other systems, etc.

2. Having established that health can indeed be considered a function system, the second section of the chapter discusses the peculiar internal structure of health systems, which shows a number of distinct partial systems: (2.1) It is explained that besides the core functional role of diagnosing and treating patients, there are a number of diverse entities performing other specific roles inside the system; (2.2) Among these entities, there is public health, which functions by communications concerned with the health and health risks of populations instead of individual patients. (2.3) The system also encompasses the presence of entities like professional councils and associations, licensing bodies, etc. with oversight, self-referential, normative, quality assurance, accredi-

---

1   The discussions in this chapter draw from diverse sources: Luhmann (1990a, 2016 and 2017a); texts on Sociology of Health and History of Medicine (Knudsen 2012 and 2015; Meyer 2015; Canguilhem 1978; Foucault 2003; Mol 2002; Vogd 2015; Bynum 2008) and several published articles on health systems.

2   A Spanish translation of the article, entitled "El código de la medicina", can be found as the fourth chapter in the book "Distinciones Directrices" published in Spain (Luhmann 2016).

tation and licensing roles; (2.4) We also find entities representing the interests and views of patients and other stakeholders receiving healthcare services. The section discusses the relations between these partial systems and their integration into a recognizable unit, the health system.

3. A discussion is then held on the complexity-reduction strategies employed in health systems. The section discusses how complexity reduction is performed in relation to the environment while the complexity of the system increases in the process.

1. Is health a function system?

In the first chapter we listed the attributes that characterize a social function system. We need to test whether those features can be found in health systems. We can start with the concept of communication. Obviously communication is central to the health system; it goes on all the time between professionals and between professionals and patients. Everything happening in a health system is communicated orally and/or in writing. Communication is so visible and constant that it is a sort of "natural" state of the system. We may even say that nothing happens, no actions are performed if some sort of communication is not announcing, or accompanying, or confirming and registering any step taken or to be taken. In a fictional scenario where communication stops, nothing could continue in the system.

In correspondence to that, the incorporation of an individual as a professional in the system is preceded by lengthy learning processes whereby the individual acquires sufficient competence in communication to be recognized as a professional of the system, in whatever role he/she might be assigned. Patients are also required, or at least expected, to communicate their complaints and confirm their understanding of the instructions given to them.

Such huge volumes of exchanges are made possible by the basic single healthy/sick binary code (a basic distinction for observations across all operations in the system). The communications are justified by assigning all that is communicated to one or the other side of the distinction. In the above-mentioned article, Luhmann notes that the sick side of the distinction is the one that leads to further communications. Healthy bodies are not of concern for the health system; the doctor shakes hands with the individual and says goodbye, sending them back into the outside environment. Health systems display the crucial feature of function systems: the deployment of a binary code in their communications.

Having established that, we can now examine whether we can see in the health sector autopoiesis as defined by Luhmann's theory. This concept holds that the system generates the means of its own reproduction, and this is done by the system alone. The reproduction of a communication-based social system is the reproduction of the communications that are system-specific, an exclusive prerogative of the system. There is no question about the fact that the health system only recognizes as its communications those generated by recognizable legitimate sources in the system. Furthermore, communications assign the potential for production of new valid communications. This way, the system communicatively controls its own, we may say, communicative reproduction.

The operational closure of function systems means that the system only works with information internally generated by itself. The system is closed for information generated outside it. This feature implies that health systems can rely exclusively on their own self-generated information. This may prompt some controversy: it could be argued, for example, that a decision by a judge in relation to provision of healthcare to privately insured patients needs to be dealt with in the health system as relevant information. In this regard, two points need to be considered. First, a function system only operates with the binary code that corresponds to it; no utterance using other binary codes is meaningful for it. The function system comprehends the universe of possible communications within that semantic sphere. However, organizations as social systems have interests in a number of different function systems; organizations have legal departments, have economic operations, have communications within the education system as well as within the science system, they interact with the media system and the political system, and so on. Organizations can do that because their unit is preserved by the exclusive principles of membership and decision-making.[3] In any organization there are specific members dealing with specific function systems, communicating through the specific code of the system in question. An organization can also communicate with other organizations because they have members who deal with matters of the same function systems; they can therefore share and use the same semantics. Operational closure is a feature of function systems; a function system cannot communicate with another function system as their

---

3   In contrast, the binary code is what preserves the unit of a function system.

semantic universes do not overlap. This may sound counter-intuitive but is of central relevance in the architecture of the theory. For the moment we can accept that health systems display operational closure, with their unique and exclusive communications often "unintelligible" to others.

Operational closure leads us to the related concept of social differentiation. As a function system only operates with the binary code that corresponds to it, no utterance using other binary codes is meaningful for it, and this is the basis of social differentiation. The differentiation separates different function systems within the society. Empirical evidence of social differentiation means it requires no further discussion. It can be easily observed. Modern societies show internal differentiations with function systems living within their own communicative spaces. The health system is one among the differentiated systems.

Two additional features that are worth mentioning at this stage are the specific programmes and the coupling with other systems. Specific programmes are linked with the binary codes; the programmes set chains of connected meanings that ultimately refer back to the founding binary code. Programmes imply logical conditional steps of selections based on true or false assertions. Health systems have plenty of exclusive programmes.

Structural coupling is the operation by which, within its operational closure, a system can observe another one and by doing that adapt its own operations, making coordination between systems possible. As an example we can think of the close mutual observation that the systems of science and of education (two distinct functional systems) engage in with the systems of health. The health system largely relies on these two systems for carrying out and improving its communications.

A simple conclusion we can take out of these sometimes controversial points is that the health function system should be understood as the unique meaning universe whereby all communications related to health and sickness are fully intelligible and understandable. We talk of the health system as a semantic dimension.

2. What is the structure of a health system?

Once we have accepted that health is a function system, we can discuss the peculiar internal structure of health systems, which shows a number of distinct sub-systems. Under the overarching frame of the health system there are several distinguishable services and functions that could not be described as generators of communications based on the healthy/sick binary code in the context of diagnosis and treatment of patients.[4]

Although healthcare delivery is at the centre of the health system and is the reason for its existence and reproduction (absorbing almost all the resources of the system), there are a number of complementary functions that play an important role in any health system, although not directly linked to the treatment of the sick.

Among those sub-systems is public health, comprehending a number of functions and communications concerned with the health of populations instead of individual patients. There are also entities with oversight, self-referential, normative and licensing roles, such as professional councils, professional associations, quality monitoring and accreditation bodies. Furthermore, we also identify entities representing the interests and views of patients and stakeholders receiving or entitled to healthcare services. We discuss each of these sub-systems next. The final task therefore is to understand how this multiplicity of sub-systems is integrated into the recognizable unit, the health system.

Under the public health banner there are numerous programmes and activities. We can for instance list: health promotion activities (including community and society-wide dissemination of health information); health surveillance; health information systems as well as related functions such as planning, monitoring and evaluation; management and implementation of health programmes such as immunization, vector controls, health surveys and risk assessments.

By looking at collective rather than individual sick patients, public health acquires a macro-perspective for self-observation of the system. Public health tries to see health as a system, distinguishing the interconnectedness and interactions the system's components develop in the process of detecting and treating patients. Using epidemiological tools, public health can observe trends, assess how the system is performing as a whole, and project scenarios.

---

4   Several texts discussing and applying the Social Systems Theory constructs (some in the health field) can be found in Knudsen and Vogd (2015), Seidl and Helge (2006), and Bakken and Hernes (2003).

The Six Pillars framework and subsequent conceptualizations such as health systems thinking, promoted by the WHO,[5] reveal the "mind set", so to speak, of the advanced public health representation of health systems. In having the capacity to represent the health system to itself, public health can also establish couplings with other systems, in attempts to "irritate" them in pursuance of advantages for the autopoiesis of the health system.

In that regard public health plays a key role in coupling with the political system to project forward health agendas. However, the representations of the health system constructed by the public health sub-system have to live with diverse representations independently constructed by each health sub-system about itself, which do not necessarily coincide or agree with the views elaborated by the public health sub-system. Still, the public health sub-system may have little influence or impact on what goes on at the core of the health system, i.e. the service provision where diagnostics and treatments are uninterruptedly delivered.

Moving on with the discussion on the sub-systems, we can now address those sub-systems with oversight, self-referential, normative and licensing roles, specifically focused on professionals.[6]

Medical as well as other professional councils, legally in charge of licensing and controlling professional authorization to practise, perform a crucial self-observation role for the health systems. The control of professional licensing is a self-regulatory competence by which the system assures the maintenance of the binary code and the integrity of the communications deploying the code in all its expanded levels of complexities (including all specialities and professional practices).

In doing this, the professional councils play a fundamental role. They are empowered by the political system, through legal instruments approved by high legislative bodies, to perform corrective and punitive actions. The councils carry out vital tasks for health systems. They also constitute models to be replicated at smaller scale at the level of health facilities and regions, which for instance acquire ethical oversight responsibilities, resorting to the higher level for more serious cases, requiring for instance suspension of licences.

---

5 *Systems Thinking for Health Systems Strengthening*, edited by Don de Savigny and Taghreed Adam (WHO 2009).

6 Surely public health also has oversight, self-referential, normative and licensing roles, however these roles focus on the health system, not the individual professions.

Furthermore, at this sub-system we can also identify professional associations interested in representing the interests of the professionals – for example, concerned with dissemination of information on new techniques among professionals, as well as training and orienting the adoption of the techniques and standards; guiding, coordinating and promoting professionals in specific fields and specialities.

To be sure, professional qualifications are undertaken in the education system, however much professional training happens in the course of the daily activities of treating patients. These are health system activities rather than of other function systems.

Still, at the level of this sub-system, we can observe organizations developing standards and sometimes carrying out assessments of conditions for quality of care and accreditation, which although located a step away from the provision of actual services, are relevant internal observers of the health system. These are not necessarily found or effective in every health system.

Finally, we can identify a fourth specific sub-system represented by the entities that are not engaged in the communicative conveyance of the healthy/sick binary code. However, they are relevant and generate valid communication in the system. Examples are patients' associations and healthcare users stakeholder groups. They communicate the experience of being classified as sick, and treated (or not) as such inside the system; these are recognized by the system as legitimate communications.

These four sub-systems are inside the health system, participating in the internal communications. They perform essential roles for health systems' autopoiesis. This roughly drafted architecture of health systems is summarized in Table 2.1.

This picture is certainly not free of controversy. Some readers may have noticed that we did not include any of the typical managerial functions as sub-systems of the health system, such as the financing, administration, human resources management, legal and political governance functions. The reason is that these areas belong to other function systems, such as the economic, political or legal. In short, their communications are not based on the healthy/sick binary code; they specifically communicate with other binary codes, even when they refer to patients and their treatment; their concerns are thus distinct. Within health systems' organizations, departments and divisions take care of such matters and communicate accordingly. Organizations are social systems with a "multi-contexturality" composition; we deal with this topic in Chapter 7.

Table 2.1 : Health social system structure

Sub-systems	Example of components
Healthcare service delivery	Hospitals, polyclinics, primary health care centres, pharmacies, clinical laboratories, etc.
Public health	Epidemiological, environmental and sanitary surveillance; preventive programmes; health information; surveys; risk assessments, etc.
Normalization and standards for professionals and practices	Councils, associations, accreditation, etc.
Patients and healthcare services users	Patients' associations, healthcare users' interest groups, etc.

Some readers might mention other institutions, such as universities, health insurance or ministries of health. A brief answer at this point is that they also belong to other function systems. Qualification of professionals is mainly conducted in the education system, even when the teaching and health system practices seem to overlap in university hospitals, where, nevertheless, it is always possible to separate what belongs strictly to the health system and what pertains to education. Health insurance organizations obviously belong and communicate within the economic system, with their operations consisting in buying and selling health services and policies. Ministries of health, as entities belonging to governments and therefore mostly concerned with and communicating on political matters, where the binary codes government/opposition or governing/governed are the key features, belong in the first instance to the political system.

We can add that educational activities are essential for the autopoiesis of the education system. Health insurance is not essential for a health system and providers pursue their autopoiesis as organization systems. And finally, health systems continue to deliver healthcare, even in countries at war and in other extreme situations when governments, ministries of health, educational institutions, insurance organizations, etc. have totally collapsed. In such contexts, essential communications characterizing a health system persist regardless of the status of those organizations where the services are provided.

3. What are the complexity issues of a health system?

As mentioned in Chapter 1, complexity is a feature of observation, not an object in itself. Complexity refers to observation capacity and the volume of elements and relations between elements that can be observed. Observers, watching either of the two sides of the system/environment distinction, can admit complexity.

Luhmann says: "we will call an interconnected collection of elements 'complex' when ... it is no longer possible to connect every element with every other element" (Luhmann 1995, p. 24). In his words "complexity is a measure for indeterminacy or lack of information. Viewed in this way, it is the information that the system lacks fully to grasp and to describe its environment (environmental complexity) or itself (system complexity)" (Luhmann 1995, pp. 27–28).

In several of his texts, Luhmann addresses the question of complexities inside the system and in the environment. The system needs to keep its internal complexity at a level that does not compromise its autopoiesis. If the system becomes internally too complex for the tools and communications it can generate, it needs to engage in complexity reduction strategies. A system that goes beyond the limits of its capacity to articulate its increasing number of sub-systems, for instance, may risk collapsing.

One may therefore ask: Why does a system increase its complexities? The more complex a system becomes, the more complex observations it can make of the environment where it lives. As the environment has limitless or, more precisely, unknown limits of the complexities of elements and relations between elements, a system is under permanent pull to increase its competences to address the known unknowns as well as finding out the potential unknown unknowns.

Such a drive to address environmental complexity may lead the system to increase internal complexities to a point where it can no longer meaningfully maintain and reproduce itself. So, systems must permanently strike balances between their internal complexities and the complexities they address in the environment

Based on Luhmann's work, Ahlemeyer (2001) proposes a definition of complexity relevant for our discussion. In correspondence to what has already been said above, he states that "Complexity is not a system operation – nothing what the system does or what happens to it. It is rather a notion of observation and description, including self-observation and self-description" (p. 27). Furthermore, he says: "A system is complex for an observer when it is neither in a state of complete order nor of complete disorder, that is to say: when it represents a mixture of redundancy and variety", where *redundancy* means repetition of patterns or patterns of variability, and *variety* means changing of patterns.

In more concrete terms, we can say that a health system facing the challenge of an outbreak of an unknown disease (such as Ebola or Covid when they initially appeared) needs to set in motion a number of sub-systems in its response. In the process, new communications will have to develop, representing the new settings, techniques and operations to be implemented. They will add complex relations that were not in place before, and the complexity of the system will consequently increase. But from then on the system should be better equipped to identify and react to such increased complexity in its environment. The system is, from its perspective, "decreasing" the complexity of the environment, while at the same time "increasing" its own complexity.

Summary of the chapter

As a concluding summary of this chapter we can say that health systems have the characteristics of function systems as described in the Social Systems Theory. Particularly, being autopoietic systems, health systems control their reproduction by means of their internal operations, i.e. their communications.

The structure of health systems incorporates a number of sub-systems around the core healthcare service delivery function. The sub-systems, with diverse contributions, play crucial roles in the self-reference and self-observation of the health system.

Finally, the theory suggests that health systems become progressively better able to address the complexities of their environment by becoming themselves more complex. In Ahlemeyer notes, "If one wants to construct a system able to deal with a high level of environmental variety, one has to provide a sufficiently high level of system variety" (Ahlemeyer 2001, loc. 886). Key for any health system strengthening initiative is the observation of how the balance between the complexity of the system and its environment is to be preserved, guaranteeing the autopoiesis of the system.

Chapter 3 – Health Systems – Methodological issues

Luhmann's Social Systems Theory departs from the traditional empirically orientated epistemology. Social systems are self-referred systems capable of self-observation. In cybernetic language (Foerster 2014), a self-referred system is "non-trivial" because, by observing itself and interpreting its own observations, the system can change links between inputs and outputs therefore remaining to a large extent unpredictable. Besides that, by consisting of communications, social systems acquire functionalities related to the peculiarities of the social phenomenon of communication. Because of these conceptual decisions, a number of careful considerations are necessary in any attempt to acquire empirical evidence of a system's attributes and operations.

This chapter addresses key methodological concerns in studying social systems. First, we discuss the methodological implications of adopting the concepts presented in Chapters 1 and 2. Second, the following sub-section makes suggestions on how the researcher's gaze can navigate the operations of a system. The final sub-section concludes with a list of methodological points for analysing health systems and their components. A conclusion of the content of the three sub-sections is presented at the end.

1. Here we discuss the implications of recognizing health systems, their sub-systems and organizations as autopoietic. There are difficulties in approaching autopoiesis, however it is at work all the time, as otherwise any biological, psychic or social system would cease to exist.

Luhmann (2013) pointed out that the concept of autopoiesis has "weak explanatory power", indicating that although it is always at work in any living system, it fundamentally comprises all operations any system carries out. All operations contribute, or ultimately are autopoiesis in the making. In its operations the systems are continuously reproducing themselves with the means they themselves produce.

He also made other relevant remarks. In his words: "Strictly speaking, nothing can be explained by means of autopoiesies" (Luhmann 2013, p. 80). He clarifies, for instance, that the hypotheses of systems development from lower to higher levels of complexity cannot be explained by autopoiesis, because it is at work, whatever the conditions in which a system operates. But he still advocates the use of the term he classifies as "meta-theory", similar to concepts that are never problematized in other science, for example what is the soul in psychology, or the social in sociology, or life in biology, and so on. "This concept gives little information concerning concrete work", Luhmann (2013, p. 31) says.

The theory therefore needs to bring in additional concepts. The notion that the system is in charge of its own reproduction is important and must be understood and kept in mind. It is also necessary to keep in mind that Luhmann speaks about communication as the only building block of social systems; and when he refers to a system's reproduction, he is talking about reproduction by the system of the communications that are distinctly constitutive of the system. In other words, systems reproduction is reproduction of the specific communications that belong to the system.

In accepting the system's autopoiesis, one has also to agree with its corollary implication that only the system can take care of and perform its own reproduction, and for that the system should be capable of self-observation and self-organization. This has epistemological as well as practical implications for how to study health systems. Among such implications, it situates external researchers (observers) on a place of very limited or no capacity for determining or influencing the reproduction of the system.

Opening a brief parenthesis here, we may acknowledge that common sense would tell us that reproduction of the health system is made possible by the health budgets the government approves or by other sources of finance. However, we need to remember that reproduction of the health system is the reproduction of its communications, which are meaningful and can only be properly engaged with and understood internally, inside the system. As an illustration, we can consider that, although a hospital is to some extent an organization operating in the economic system and therefore performing buying and selling operations, such operations do not interfere with or become themes in the communications concerned with health and sickness and the diagnostics and treatments being performed. The two semantic universes do not, so to speak, overlap. The price of the examinations and medications does not change the considerations about how correct or wrong a diagnosis was. This example illustrates why the reproduction of what is at the core of the health system does not depend on the size of the budget. Social Systems Theory reminds us that the closure and internal generation of information is meaningful for the system.

Coming back to autopoiesis, having in mind that the observation of social systems is also second-order observation (i.e. observation of observers who are themselves able to observe and self-observe), the researchers need to be clear about who observes whom, and to be explicit about the distinction used for making observations. Observations are carried out with distinctions and therefore the observer needs to be critical about them and respective blind spots. All distinctions, and consequently all observations, have unavoidable blind spots.

Furthermore, orientating observation towards communications and what is possible to be communicatively achieved by those who communicate inside the system, the observer needs to understand how communication works. This point is further expanded in the subsequent paragraphs.

2. If a health system is observed as a function system made up of communications, the system is nowhere specifically and at the same time it is everywhere that recognized legitimate health communications take place. Therefore, researchers need to understand they are looking for an object that has a special ontological nature. The research does not need to look for buildings, equipment, physical assets or institutions. It must look for the communications deploying the healthy/sick codes inherent in all health communications, in correspondence with observations made from one or the other side of that distinction.

In line with that, it might sound counter-intuitive that ministries of health, as pointed out in the previous chapter, may only partially belong to the health system; or rather, to a large extent, a ministry is part of the political system. It all depends on the nature and codes of communication circulating inside a ministry of health. Nevertheless, the researcher may also find many organizations operating with the codes of the health system, coupled with other organizations and systems identified as relevant for their autopoiesis.

In short, communication is the key element for understanding systems. A good grasp of the recursive nature of communication (it is always possible to communicate about communication), and three components of communication – content, utterance and understanding – is therefore necessary. Furthermore, as all communications are based on language, the possibility of "yes" or "no" is always present, meaning that any communication, either accepting or rejecting what has been communicated, can interlace subsequent communications. And finally, we need to recognize the importance of double contingencies, i.e. the selections made by each side while communicating. Communications include oral and written forms.

An important challenge is related to the fact that communications also imply the possibility of communication about communication. This extraordinary evolutionary achievement of communication creates a vast potential for recursive self-reference. The incorporation of self-reference in empirical studies represents a considerable difficulty which the traditional approaches to empirical observations do not deal with. Self-reference refers both to the system's capacities and to the observers' positions.

3. Wrapping up what was discussed in the previous sections, we summarize the methodological orientation derived from Luhmann's theory. The points below give a draft conception of the methodological approaches that can guide the researcher.

3.1 It is important to take the perspective that health systems are autopoietic.

3.2 It is necessary to start with a clear identification of what are the actual autopoietic units the researchers are approaching in their studies, and whether they are only small components of a larger autopoietic unit, whether they have any degree of autonomy for controlling communication and therefore continuing their autopoiesis. Autopoiesis necessarily implies production of one system's means of reproducing its communications. Here an understanding of the two types of social system is required; the researchers should know whether they want to address the health system as a differentiated overarching *function system* of the society (based on its specific binary code), or rather as specific *organizations* operating in a circumscribed manner, with clear membership criteria and decision-making structures.

3.3 The approach highlights the need to acknowledge *operational closure*, which implies that the system observes its environment and transforms observations into information inside the system. Only information generated by the system can then be meaningfully communicated inside it. In its closure, the system uses its specific binary code to determine whether the internally generated information is or is not relevant for the system.

3.4 In particular, for the organizations that are recognized as part of the health system, membership and decision-making are defining bases for organizations' closure. Organizations pursue their autopoiesis with those identified as members and the decisions they take (decisions are recognized as such once they are communicated).

3.5 The approach also emphasizes the need to locate the observer; researchers must be aware of where they stand, whether inside or outside the system they are studying, and whether they are carrying out first- or second-order observation, meaning observing observers or even observing observers observing themselves. Awareness of the unavoidability of blind spots is also needed.

3.6 With clarity about both the observation position and the autopoietic self-referential and operationally closed nature of the systems being observed, the researchers should be able to make critical judgement of the purpose of the investigation and the possibilities of having the results (conclusions and recommendations) considered by the organizations being studied.

3.7 Therefore, when choosing themes for carrying out empirical observation, the researchers should be aware that the findings exist within an autopoietic, operationally closed communication-based system that makes selections. The researchers also need to consider that the communications that will be produced by the research may find easy acceptance in the social system of science, where the researchers may come from, but may not be entirely recognized as relevant for the health system in focus. The two systems, health and science, operate with distinctively different sets of codes and communications programmes.

3.8 A system, defined in opposition to its environment and essentially composed by communications, should be approached having in mind that it is constantly selecting and reproducing communications in line with previous communications and decisions, and with the potential to encompass the subsequent ones.

3.9 Clarity on the nature of internal communications constitutive of the system is essential; this means observation of those communicating and the channels of communications, with clear understanding of directionality, expectations, recursive possibilities and the contingent nature (meaning the possibility to be different). Communications can be "mapped", "inventoried" or somehow reflected in the descriptions of the systems, but cannot be exhausted. As part of the autopoiesis of the system, communications are always being generated and kept open for new topics and formulations.

3.10 Finally, researchers need to pay attention to the possibilities that observed organizations may enter into structural coupling with other organizations, allowing for mutual influences, while maintaining their individual closure. Luhmann (2013, p. 88) talks about a system "irritating" or being "irritated" by other systems, meaning a system (organizations included) can observe another system and in consequence of those observations produce internal information that once processed can also be observed by the other system. In this process, the two systems, preserving their operational closure, can still observe each other and that can result in coordination. Of particular relevance, if the research includes policy and political themes, the researchers should be aware of the ways the political system operates in contrast with the health system and its organizations, and understand how the coupling between these two function systems is possible, as mutual observation.

Summary of the chapter

To conclude, Luhmann has been criticized (see Chapter 8) for having not conducted empirical data collection to confirm the validity of his concepts. Luhmann's work is entirely developed in the space of theoretical reflection, although informed by concrete observation of the social reality. Therefore, for many, there is no clear prescription on empirical methods to be deployed in fieldworks. However, these judgements do not decrease the value of what the theory offers for reflection and understanding of the operations of social systems, and the actions and interventions that can be derived from them. Empirical works and methodological approaches are therefore territories open for innovation and creativity. Of relevance, perhaps, is to consider that research is mostly conducted in the social systems of science or education (two different social systems), and health systems operate within different semantic orders. The reader will find more discussions on this topic throughout the chapters, with some more specific reflections in the final remarks chapter.

Chapter 4 – Health Systems Thinking and Social Systems Theory

In the last decade a lot of studies have been published under the banner of health systems strengthening or health systems thinking (HST). A Medline search using the term "health systems strengthening" finds 7804 articles from 2010 to 2021, an average of 650 articles per year. The search using "health systems thinking" gives 8324 hits (yearly average of 694) for the same period. This indicates the high relevance health systems themes have acquired. Acknowledging such prominent attention to the topic, in this chapter health systems thinking approaches are critically assessed in the light of Luhmann's theory of social systems.

In simple terms, health systems thinking is an attempt to bring together two sets of knowledge: on one side, the understanding of the characteristic attributes of health sectors, with their huge diversity of elements and relations (practices, diagnostics, treatments, technologies, specializations, stakeholders, structures, organizations, programmes, policies and so on); and on the other side, systems theories, with a plethora of approaches, methods and tools from diverse scientific fields. The chapter raises the question that a lot is not granted in the attempt to link these two universes. While the notion of a health system implies an acceptance of its mosaic-like outlook, without conceptualizing the gathering of parts of systems into a distinguishable unit, there is also a leap of faith in accepting methods and tools used in other fields (a collection resembling a *bricolage* itself), believing they offer the means to understand the nature of any health system.

The wide-ranging notions identified by HST as distinctive attributes of health systems include a number of features which are not interrelated or integrated into a comprehensive articulated whole. Among those notions of systems' characteristics we can list self-organization, constant changes, control by feedback loops, complex dynamics and non-linearity, time lags between inputs and outcomes, resistance to change, historical dependence, critical stakeholders and contextual influences, policies and actions generating counter-intuitive and unpredictable effects, etc. (WHO 2009).

Definitions of health systems thinking related to tools and methods says that systems thinking is "a way to view the world using the general logic underlying various systems theory (e.g. general systems theory, chaos theory or complexity theory), informed by a wide range of relevant tools and methods (e.g. systems dynamics, modelling, structured conceptualization, or network analysis), the choice of which will largely depend on the question at hand, the context and available capacity" (Adam and de Savigny 2012).

The tools imported from other fields include boundary critique, soft systems methodology, critical systems heuristics, sense-making frameworks for problems, causal loop diagrams, social network analysis, human systems dynamics, process mapping, modelling systems dynamics, scenario techniques, outcome mapping, and so on (de Savigny et al. 2017). Harmonization and compatibility of all these notions, tools and approaches has not been attempted. Health systems thinking, as a knowledge territory, is therefore a patchwork of unrelated techniques and concepts. One is left with the impression that, lacking precise understanding of what a health system is, the field is open to absorb any tool from any scientific field that seems to help to fill the void.

As mentioned above, this merging of these two universes (health sector features and systems thinking tools) indeed remains a matter of good intention. The lack on both sides of a unifying theoretical body, which could help, on one hand, to visualize health systems' unit and, on the other, to see the combined validity of the tools to approach this rather multi-faceted object, is a major weakness of the health systems thinking endeavour. This chapter suggests that Luhmann's theory may contribute to overcome that deficit.

The discussion in this chapter therefore addresses the features presented as characteristic of health systems in the text *Health Systems, for Health Systems Strengthening* published in 2009 by the World Health Organization's Alliance for Health Policy and Systems Research.[1] Below, the systemic features identified by HST are listed and questions are raised. The second section of the chapter offers answers in line with Social Systems Theory perspectives.

---

1   This text has become the key reference in the domain of health systems thinking, with the characterization echoed in many subsequent works.

Questions

1. *Systems are resistant to change and systems are always changing* – How can researchers know at what measure they are dealing with resistance to change or with change itself? How can they distinguish whether they are looking at something that is changing or something that is resisting change, or indeed something that is doing both at the same time? And how about changes in the way the system resists change? Can these still count as resistance or change?
2. *Systems are governed by feedback loops* – When does a feedback loop have to be discontinued, modified, incremented, replaced, etc.? A stubborn feedback loop certainly leads any system to collapse. Something has to govern the feedback loop for the sake of achieving the system's objectives; what controls the feedback loop? Furthermore, how can governance dynamics be translated and analysed in terms of causal loops, when they often involve complex non-repetitive decision-making processes, which cannot be described as automated mechanisms?
3. *Systems are comprised of networks of nodes and ties, and networks take defining structures* – A number of questions can be raised in relation to systems and networks. How is the network's nodes and ties behaviour determined by the structure of the network when that structure itself is brought about by the behaviour of its nodes and ties? Is this a recursive phenomenon or just a tautology? How can a network incorporate changes into itself and respond to changes in the environment, and what drives it to do so? Will change unavoidably lead to the demise of the network in its current structure? How can this be predicted? A major weakness of the network theory seems to be its lack of incorporation of changing dynamics and factors.
4. *Systems are made of tightly linked parts, and changes in one are likely to have unforeseen effects in the other parts of the system* – Luhmann (2013) argues that complete interconnectedness and interdependence of all a system's elements is highly improbable. If that were the case, he says, all disturbance would require the entire system to be rebalanced anew; that would take a long time and would consume precious energy. It is therefore necessary to consider that the commonly held view of the integration of the system does not correspond to reality, and systems in fact develop internal specialized reactions and capabilities to isolate disturbances and solve them separately. The question should then be reformulated as how far a system separates or integrates its parts, and how vulnerable/resilient it might become in con-

sequence of that. What is better? To have tight internal connectedness or a certain degree of looseness, with parts performing adjustments independently? These are questions usually raised in relation to decentralization.

5. *Systems are counter-intuitive, have large numbers of elements interacting in non-linear fashion, and therefore have cause–effect relationships that may not be fully knowable* – That seems to be a reasonable understanding, supported by a non-explicit notion that complexity may include known unknowns as well as unknown unknowns. However, if that notion is adopted as valid, there are a number of implications to be considered. How can a system function within its own complexity? How can a complex system still operate effectively and reproduce itself? What can systems do that researchers, with their definition of complexity, cannot observe? Should the conclusion be that systems know better about themselves than what the researchers can actually figure out about them?

6. *Systems are path-dependent, meaning they have a history and the history influences behaviour* – In this style of formulation, the statement cannot be contested. However, the statement also opens a universe of questions. How can that come about? From the history of a system, what is forgotten? And how does what is maintained acquire the capacity to affect the present behaviour of the system? Of the countless things that happen to and in a system, how does it separate what is relevant for the future from what should be left behind? Do systems have selective memory? If so, how does it operate?

7. *Systems have boundaries but their boundaries are impossible or very difficult to know with precision* – The theme of systems' boundaries is a recurrent one and also one that leads to considerable misunderstandings. What sort of boundaries do systems have? Physical? Logical? Semantic? What do the boundaries separate? A system's components from non-components? How can the non-components still relevant for the system be distinguished from those the system should not care about? What are the criteria and processes to separate them? Furthermore, how does the system maintain its boundaries and ensure they are effective?

8. *Systems are self-organizing – system dynamics arise spontaneously from internal structures* – This statement is also often used; however, little is explained about how this happens to be the case. If systems are indeed self-organizing, it is necessary to identify the "self" that organizes itself; where is it? Self-organization implies a number of capabilities and functionalities; the system should be able to make distinctions, observe, observe itself, choose selection criteria, make selections, decide about what to do with whatever

is selected, find a coherent fit with previous selections, and so on. The self has to have all these competences and much more. It also has to deal with what is outside the system, as for instance other systems in the spheres of politics, the law, education, science, and so on. How does such a "self" appear, and how does it consistently deal with all of that? Or is this self only a metaphor?

As this large number of questions shows, the tasks of health systems thinking and the use of the suggested tools are endeavours full of uncertainties. A message this book conveys about the health systems thinking approach and its dominance in health systems research is of its recognizable value, but also the need to move forward, adopting more consistent theoretical references.

Answers

The points below present tentative answers to the questions raised in the previous section. They briefly discuss each of the key features that proponents of health systems thinking have promoted. To make it easier for the reader to connect the answers to the respective questions, those questions are summarized at the start of each paragraph.

1. *Systems are resistant to change and systems are always changing* – How can researchers know to what extent they are dealing with resistance to change or with change itself? How can they distinguish whether they are looking at something that is changing or something that is resisting change, or even something that is doing both at the same time? And how about changes in the way the system resist changes? Can these still count as resistance or change? More than a play on words, the critical intention is to emphasize that without a comprehensive theoretical framework the researcher is likely to get lost. If, as Luhmann indicates, systems pursue their autopoiesis, then resistance and change can be interpreted from a clearer perspective. Change or resistance become meaningful in the context of the autopoiesis of the system; with these considerations, the analysis has a better sense of direction. Change happens when the system observes the potential advantages of answering the demands better, reflecting the pressures observed in the external as well as internal environment. In contrast, resistance to change would be a process of preserving the integrity

of the system as it is operating, avoiding the risk of depleting the system of its capacity to process and respond to the internal and perceived external pressures; the system would have the paramount orientation to preserve its capacity to observe, process and decide what to do next, whether retaining redundant elements or incorporating new ones. Nothing other than the autopoiesis of the system is at stake.

2. *Systems are governed by feedbacks loops* – when does a feedback loop have to be discontinued, modified, increased, replaced, etc.? A stubborn feedback loop will certainly lead to the collapse of the system. Something has to govern the feedback loops for the sake of reaching systems' functions; the pursuit of autopoiesis aims cannot itself be carried out by feedback loops. What is governing the loops then? Luhmann's conceptualization of recurring communications, which maintains but also changes and adjusts themes, codes, programmes and expectations (remaining open to additional meanings), is more suitable than the concept of feedback loops with its mechanical outlook. A self-organizing system can choose which loops to set in motion, interrupt or discontinue; in this way, instead of governing, the loops are governed upon.

3. *Systems are comprised of networks of nodes and ties, and networks take defining structures* – How is the behaviour of the network's nodes determined by the structure of the network when the network structure itself is brought about by the behaviour of its nodes and ties? If this is a recursive phenomenon, repeating itself again and again, behaviour–structure–behaviour–structure–behaviour–structure, and so on, what prevents the system from getting into a pattern that will never change and therefore will never incorporate any responses to changes in the environment? Will that unavoidably lead to the demise of the system? The way out of this conundrum seems to be in the self-referring and self-organizing capabilities of the systems. The Systems Theory indicates that the system can observe the operation of the internal and external networks. The self-observation allows the system to decide on the patterns of the network that may need to be changed. A network that cannot be observed and cannot be adjusted, whatever the observational capability, cannot belong to the system itself. Although the self-observation is carried out by elements of the internal network, the communications that such self-observations entail are not predicted or directed by the structure of the network. Communications construct and change networks, not the other way round (see additional discussion on Networks in Chapter 5 on health systems thinking tools).

4. *Systems are made up of tightly linked sub-systems and a change in one may affect the others* – Luhmann argues that complete interconnectedness and interdependence of all a system's elements is a highly improbable state. According to him, if that were the case, all disturbances would require the entire system to be rebalanced anew; taking time and consuming precious energy. He said that, while the system tries to rebalance, another disturbance may occur and the system could be severely burdened, never achieving a stable state. For that reason, it is necessary to consider that the commonly held view of the integration of the system does not correspond to reality. As an evolutionary characteristic of systems, they in fact developed internal specialized reactions and capabilities to isolate disturbances and solve them separately. The question should then be reformulated as how far a system integrates its parts and how vulnerable it might become in consequence of that. What is then better: a system with tight internal connectedness or degrees of looseness? Empirical studies aiming to answer such a question should give up on the old conceptions of tight interconnectedness of all a system's elements.

5. *Systems are counter-intuitive, have large numbers of elements interacting in non-linear fashion, and therefore have cause–effect relationships that may not be fully knowable* – That seems a reasonable understanding, that complexity may include known unknowns as well as unknown unknowns. However, how can a system function with its own complexity? Should the conclusion be that systems know better about themselves than what the researchers can actually figure out about them? If that argument puts the researchers in a humble (most likely realistic) position, it is still, on the other hand, necessary to have an explanatory model to give an account of the way the system deals with its own complexity and the elements unknown to the researchers. How can a system, with its complexity, still operate adequately and reproduce itself? What can systems do that researchers, with their definition of complexity, cannot work out? If the non-apprehensible reality of systems is a matter of fact, what are the implications for those studying and working inside them? Will they have to admit their limitations from the start? Will they have to accept that the system knows better? The notion that systems have self-organizing capabilities helps to put most of these questions in a better perspective, and perhaps answer some of them. Self-organization requires a number of related functions (point 8 expands this topic).

6. *Systems are path-dependent, meaning they have a history and the history influences the current behaviour* – The statement opens a universe of questions. How can that come about? From the history of a system, what is forgotten and how does what is maintained affect the present behaviour? Of the countless things happening to and in a system, how does it separate what is relevant for the future from what should be left behind? Do systems have selective memory? If so, how does it operate? These are all pertinent questions triggered by the statement. Two points from the Social Systems Theory help in addressing these questions. One is about the complexity reduction capabilities of the system. Systems face huge complexities in their environment but can only deal with a limited number of elements they can observe in the environment. This operation reduces complexities (of what the system observes).[2] Besides that, once external elements become information inside the system, the system also needs to keep the internal complexity-enhancing possibilities under control (to avoid the risk of self-destruction). In this way, a system constructs its history and maintains the memory of the internal and external advances it is constantly making. However, disappointments occur, and expectations about both the internal performance and the external observed elements are actualized in unpredictable ways. That forces the system to constantly find a balance between keeping redundant elements and trying innovation. In one or the other case, the system should make its choices for the sake of its autopoiesis.
7. *Systems have boundaries but their boundaries are impossible or very difficult to know with precision* – The theme of systems' boundaries is a recurrent one. What sort of boundaries does a system have? Physical? What do the boundaries separate? A system's components from its non-components? If yes, what are the criteria to separate them? In particular, how far can an internal network stretch itself and still include external nodes and ties that can be considered part of the system? Where are the lines identifying those to be considered outsiders, despite them having ties with inside nodes?

---

2   As Annemarie Mol says about numerical measurements for diagnosis of vascular problems, for instance, "walking distances without pain in the legs": "Once numbers are scribbled in the patient's file, they come to have an independent existence as 'indicators', and possible errors of translation are no longer retrievable. Nor is the tone of voice (confident, hesitant, pleading). Thus some complexities are left out" (Mol 2002, p. 221). The reduction of complexities thus achieved is fundamental for proceeding with the clinical exploration to reach a final diagnosis.

Furthermore, how does the system maintain its boundaries and ensure they are effective? This list of questions already indicates how tricky the boundary issue is and how difficult it is to tackle these points without a comprehensive model of what is inside and outside a system and how these limits can be drawn. The Social Systems Theory takes a radical perspective in that regard. Systems are made up of communications; therefore the boundaries are not physical. What differentiates one system from another is the set of communications a system recognizes as belonging to it, in contrast with the others that are observed as belonging to other systems or the environment. The legal system would not make a diagnosis of a patient because it does not communicate in those terms; in the same way a health system will never make a decision characterizing a certain occurrence as legal or illegal. Each system communicates within the frame of its own binary codes. Meanings and no other type of separation make boundaries. Organizations, as a type of social system, also draw their boundaries with meanings and communications – in this case, communications based on the decisions taken in the organizations (which are carried out by those indicated by the membership criteria; members and non-members know their status vis-à-vis the organizations by the communications they maintain within it). The second key point is operational closure. The system is communicatively closed but observationally open; this means a system can only communicate internally (with the exception of organizations; see Chapter 7), but can observe the environment and the other systems in it. The information used in communications has to be produced internally. The environment does not have information. Information is the internal elaboration of what the system has observed in its environment. The same way that no one can have their own thoughts running in someone else's mind. These two points, operational closure and the demarcation by meanings and communications, set the question about boundaries on a more promising ground.

8. *Systems are self-organizing – system dynamics arise spontaneously from internal structures* – This statement is often used; however, little is explained about how this happens to be the case (the *advanced topics* in the Annex has a section on *System's Self-Reference*, expanding this important topic of the theory). If systems are indeed self-organizing, it is necessary to find the "self" that organizes itself: where is it? Furthermore, self-organizing implies a number of capabilities and functionalities; for instance, the system should be able to draw distinctions, observe, observe itself, choose selection cri-

teria, make selections, decide about what to do with whatever is selected, insert the selection in a coherent fit with previous selections, and so on. The self has to have all these competences and much more. How does such a "self" come about? Social Systems Theory says that all is done communicatively. Communication is the basis for self-reference and ultimately the autopoiesis of a system. Through the recursive essential nature of communication, by which the parts involved in it can retroactively refer to what had been communicated and then subsequently move on to confirming (or not) the understanding of the messages received, communication and its memories can be the bases for systemic self-reflection and self-reference. Self-organizing, according to the theory, is carried out internally by a system's own communicative competences. The role of communication – with its inherent recursive nature – for the construction of any system cannot be overemphasized. Self-organization does not arise spontaneously or randomly, as casual arrangements of parts that eventually become functional. Indeed, no system should leave its self-organization to chance. Self-organization needs to be understood in the context of autopoiesis, as operations by which the system seeks to reproduce its operational communicative capabilities, according to what the system evaluates as essential for its survival and preservation of its identity. Identity is communicatively constructed. Self-organization is one of those concepts that can easily be thrown into a discussion about characteristics of systems but is quite tricky when comes to explaining its mechanisms, and even more so in observing how it comes about.

Summary

We try here to bring together the discussions from the two preceding sections, with inputs from previous chapters, and draw some conclusions. The reflection starts with the perception that, in Health Systems Thinking, *systems* appear as collections of possible attributes and functionalities, with many elements and relations not yet grasped in their totality and complexity.

In the face of the enormity of the scientific challenge to unpack and repack health systems in some coherent unit keeping systemic features together, the WHO's tentative initial steps consisted in promoting a framework to assist those assessing, organizing and managing health systems. In 2007, the WHO published the Six Pillars framework. According to that framework, the system is supported by or is itself those Six Pillars. If anyone wanted to approach a health system as such, attention was to be given to all the pillars, which represented differentiated spaces of practices, expertise, inputs and outputs that one could find in any health system. The approach recommended a balance of attention and support to the pillars. None of them or their interactions should be neglected, the guide prescribed.

For all those schooled in organizational and managerial matters for the last 60 years or so, that was an obvious call. The organization of an enterprise has to comprehend sets of functions that individually have some independence concerning their own objectives, but at the same time are highly reliant on each other. The advice that the system cannot reach its expected results if the basic components are not taken into account could hardly come as a surprise. In one way or another, as for any type of business, the Six Pillars correspond to sets of basic components of any public or private health enterprise.[3]

Health systems thinking therefore appeared subsequently as an attempt to advance to the next level – the "state of the art", so to speak – which nevertheless so far has consisted of a collection of bits and pieces, like in a mosaic.

For HST, the underlying notion is that a system has a number of elements (nodes) linked to each other by ties (relations), which jointly make up a network. A network has a certain structure that explains and determines and is determined by the behaviour of the nodes and ties. Besides that, the system shows regularity in the way the links between the nodes follow sequential possibly stable patterns, the so-called processes. These processes are repeated and maintained in an expected consistent fashion. Some processes and links seem to gather in clusters with some peculiar circularity causation, where effects determine causes, causes determine effects and so on, in loops that keep running with presumed stability.

Besides these features, the system also has an apparent capability to change these internal dispositions; the term learning and adaptation is used to characterize the occurrence of changes. Ideas of multiple simultaneous causality, non-linearity, indeterminacy and unpredictability are also tentatively incorporated into the efforts of conceiving health systems. This implies

---

3   The Six Pillars framework conceives of health systems as comprised of: 1) medicines, vaccines and other technologies; 2) health information; 3) health service delivery; 4) health workforce; 5) leadership and governance; and 6) financing. If we remove the word health (and closely related words like vaccines and medicines) from the names of these items, the list can be applied to any kind of business.

that changes in a certain arrangement in the system can have consequences far beyond the immediately recognizable close connections; the effects could happen well into the future or into some other dispositions apparently independent from the changed ones, although belonging to the same system.

This is not the end. Health systems thinking is further enriched with additional features. It defends that systems also have boundaries, although the nature, location or constitution of those limits are not precisely established. These boundaries, whatever they are, nevertheless do not seem to lock or isolate the system inside itself. Boundaries are accepted as possibly porous and allow things in and out, permitting relationships between whatever is outside the system and something allegedly inside. How inside and outside remain where they are and do not get confused about their locations is not fully addressed.

This collection of elements and functionalities is still supposed to be kept together in some operationally consistent manner by a self-organizing capability. Systems are supposed to know how to organize themselves. The health system is expected to be doing this, and be improving its adaptation and development as a result of that. Whether self-organizing capabilities are spontaneous, automatic processing competences, an inevitable outcome of the natural interlocking of the components of the system interacting with each other, or have all of those as well as other origins, is not clear. Self-organization is kept as a matter of "belief", or perhaps the attribution of managers of the system, whoever they might be, with a tacit understanding that as long as the researchers keep looking, something will appear more clearly out of this mosaic-like collection of elements.

Social System Theory brings to the debate a set of concepts that can put the pieces of the health system together in a more comprehensive and consistent way. Health systems pursue their autopoiesis; they do that by reproducing the communications they have the prerogative to make; they have boundaries established by the specific meanings they use; they can observe themselves, other systems and the environment; by doing so and communicating internally they show self-reference and self-organizing competences; by performing self-observation and self-organization, the system can manage its own complexity by the selection capabilities of communications themselves.

The next chapter continues the debate with critical reflections on tools currently used under the banner of "Health Systems Thinking", as described in the book *Applied Systems Thinking for Health Systems Research, a Methodological Handbook*, edited by D. de Savigny, K. Blanchet and T. Adam (2017).

Chapter 5 – Health Systems Thinking Tools and Social Systems Theory

Key texts in the health systems thinking literature do acknowledge that tools are simplifying ways of addressing complexities. Tools ignore elements of complex realities to focus on a few of them, about which the tools can offer complexity-reducing models.

As is always the case in relation to models and modelling, they narrow down the fields of observation and provide reduced portrayals of reality. That is unavoidable. Researchers are aware of these limitations. Nevertheless, they justifiably believe the tools used will yield results that can be of use.

That is the main point of discussion in this chapter. The reduction of complexity thus achieved may deeply undermine the comprehensive understanding of what health systems in fact are. The tools selected for discussion are described in the book edited by D. de Savigny, K. Blanchet and T. Adam (2017). They are:

- Network analysis
- Boundary critique
- Process mapping
- Causal loop diagrams

Before discussing the selected four examples of tools promoted by health systems thinking, a reflection on the relation between the science system and the health system may contribute to the comprehension of what is discussed next.

5.1 Scientific systems observing health systems

Health system thinking tools were developed and primarily belong to the science system, a function system with the same characteristics of operational closure, autopoiesis and, in this case, orientation with the true/false binary code (true and false being the two sides of a distinction used to value models, explanations, theories, hypotheses, evidence, etc. communicated in the system). The efforts to apply the tools and find the value to be attached to the results yielded by them are the communicative work of the function system of science.

HST tools are therefore used inside the science system to observe health systems. The same tools were and are applied to other systems (economic system, education system, etc.). The science system is concerned with developing, testing and confirming the results of the tools, validating them with the true/false code. For the science system, the health system is external and belongs to the environment. The science system cannot interfere with or operate inside the health system; only the health system itself can operate inside itself.

This is what the Social Systems Theory says. No matter how big the effort to observe and measure characteristics of the health system, scientific observations will still be done from outside the health system. The health system already has many ways of observing itself. It must do so because its self-observations are vital for its autopoiesis and cannot be delegated to or borrowed from outsiders, no matter the accuracy and good intentions of the science system. As said, the codes and orientations adopted by each of the two systems are different. Cross-systems communications are not possible, although mutual observation and irritation can and do occur. The coupling of the two systems gives the impression that information seems to be circulating from one system to another; however that cannot happen, according to Luhmann's theory.

Possibly, many health systems find the results of the use of HST tools useful for their own self-observation and related decisions. But the health system will be the final judge of the usefulness and applicability of the findings. This cannot be different. The two systems are independent sovereign domains; not sovereign by decree or legal enforcement; sovereign for the impossibility of autopoiesis of a system being taken care of by another system, and for the impossibility of communications from one system becoming communications of another system. This would be like someone's thoughts being inserted into someone else's consciousness. This is an absolute impossibility in Luhmann's world. Consciousness operates under the same "law" of operational closure, and there cannot be direct communication from one consciousness to another; all communications are social and all coupling of consciousnesses is achieved through the social, as long as the two observe each other.

It is therefore important to recognize the limitations of the acquisition and applicability of knowledge. More importantly, the impossibility for the science system to meaningfully reproduce the entire health system inside the science system itself has to be accepted as an unavoidable limitation in dealing with complexities (be it in the environment, in the system being observed from outside, or in the system that observes itself). No system is able to perform such a task in relation to any other system, because none of them have what is technically called the *requisite variability*, or wealth of descriptive constructs and observational capabilities, to address the complexities of another system.

Instead, the science system directs its attention to limited specific sections of the health system to which it can apply its tools. Out of these applications, some specific descriptions of details of the health system are produced, while the totality of the health system will remain well beyond the grasp of the specific tool the science system chooses to use. Indeed, the science system has no illusions about the limitations of the findings.

Process mapping, causal loop diagrams, social network analysis, boundary critique and critical system heuristics, and any of the other tools, will not overcome the incommensurability of the two systems. There will always be gaps that cannot be bridged, where a system will remain opaque or unobservable to the other.

The scientists can still continue investing time, money and brainpower in teasing out, improving the existing tools, and developing new ones. But the perspective of limitations cannot be erased. The operational closure, under which function systems operate, the health systems and the science systems alike, cannot be dismissed. Investigation results useful for the health system are only those the health system itself can recognize as such, according to its own references.

Scientific careers can still be built and developed around the ideas of dissecting the health system and finding out its secrets, attempting to get to its inner nature. As in the seventeenth and eighteenth centuries, the advance of the knowledge of human anatomy promised to give the power to heal all diseases. When the work was done, the physiology instead became the holder of the secrets of eternal health. And so on; since then, many other scientific fields have opened up to explore the secrets of the human body: anatomo-physiology, pathology, biochemistry, molecular biology, each digging into many specific specialities such as immunology, neurology, etc. Those studying health systems should however understand that they are approaching an autopoietic entity already performing its self-observations as opposed to the unawareness of, for instance, the anatomy, in relation to itself.

Taking a short detour to add complementary reflections on this point, a research programme could try to trace the appearance of the tools and their use for detecting features of health systems. It can be expected that these tools were designed and planned within academic institutions, i.e. inside the science system. The investigation could address the hypothesis that health systems did not take the initiative to develop such tools for making self-descriptions. If this hypothesis is correct, the health system became an object of scientific investigation by the interests mobilized within the science system. One could conclude that the science system is concerned to convince itself that it has the conceptual and methodological resources to approach the health system and construct narratives about it, with internal scientific validation.

The science system fulfils its functions of communicating truthful matters, based on rigorous programmes of methods and analysis. The validation reverberates in the reproduction of publications on the same topic, adopting the same conceptual frames and methods, and the reappearance of the same contents in academic production of undergraduate, masters and doctoral essays and dissertation theses. The reproduction reinforces the validation processes, further legitimates the contents, the authors and the narratives, and that is all the science system needs in order to perform its autopoiesis.

The health system may observe, with high, low or no interest, what is happening in the science system. Where the coupling between the two systems has been working for endeavours the two may be taking together (developing new drugs, new technologies, new organizational arrangements, new programmes, etc.), it is possible that additional couplings come about with the intention of performing studies or implementing changes for example in line with what the HST tools may have suggested. Regardless of what the opportunities for such couplings entail or favour, the calculation the health system makes concerns its own autopoiesis, not the autopoiesis of the science system. Such calculations have to convincingly indicate the advantages the health system will obtain. It is therefore important that the observers outside the health system, i.e. the researchers themselves, reflect on the way the health system will see the results of the investigations carried out with the chosen tools.

Questions such as "how does the identification of the social network that exists at the moment among those implementing such and such programmes help the system in achieving its goals?" may or may not be formulated. Of course scientists do think and strategize about the chances of project acceptance, and try to sell their work as best they can; but the health system will be judging it from its own perspective, which to a great extent is beyond the full grasp of the scientist. It might be boring to repeat this, but one should never lose sight of the fact that there are two different function systems, no matter that one may consider the apparent advantages of their coupling to be evident.

Having said that, the following reflections on the HST tools look into the specifics of each of these tools taken as examples. The overall understanding exposed in the last paragraphs touched upon the common perspective by which all tools can be judged in reference to the fact that they belong to the science system in the first place. Let's now discuss the four examples.

5.2 Network analysis

References to networks as a basic element constitutive of systems are present throughout the HST literature. However, there is little discussion on the relations between networks and systems. In fact Social Systems Theory and Networks Theory are two separate branches of sociological thinking that do not agree with each other in many respects. The explicit acceptance of networks as part of the health system would meet protest and requests for qualifications from both sides of the contest.

However, Luhmann's theory offers the conceptual arsenal to address the topic,[1] helping to clarify the role of networks in relation to systems. First, it is necessary to be clear that networks are not systems in the way the Social Systems Theory understands them. Networks are not autopoietic nor present operational closure, key conceptual notions to characterise systems according to Social Systems Theory.

In a good-humoured encounter between Graham Norton (philosopher, proponent of object-orientated ontology) and Bruno Latour (social scientist, known as the Prince of the Networks and a prominent reference for networks as a sociological construct), transcribed in a book called *The Prince and the Wolf* (2011), Graham stated that the weakness of the conceptualization of networks

---

[1] Readers are referred to "Luhmann's Systems Theory and Network Theory", by M. Bommes and V. Tack (2006), for a thorough discussion on networks and Social Systems Theory.

is the fact that considering an object as defined by the relations it establishes with others cannot account for changes.

According to Graham, a network is studied and portrayed at a given moment, but what happens between one moment and the next cannot be explained by the network theory. Such criticism can be raised of any attempt to describe health systems as networks, and users of Social Network Analysis (SNA) are in fact aware of this shortcoming. Yes, networks can be described at two different moments in time, the differences can be identified, but the process of becoming different and the dynamic factors behind it are not explained or foreseen by the theory. The most one can arrive at with SNA is a limited picture of the relations between nodes established by ties, without being able to indicate what would happen next. The theory does not explain what in the nodes or in the ties or in both lead to dynamics that can produce changes in the network. Whether a certain node or a particular tie is established or not, is effective or not, goes beyond the explanatory capacity of the theory. Still, this is a critic of network analysis, which does not include the Systems Theory perspective; we get into that next.

From the Systems Theory perspective, a number of points are not properly taken into account. First is the recursive nature of communication, the contingence by which selections are made and then communicated, triggering new communications that may sustain or reject what has been previously said, and therefore the unavoidability of uncertainties (and need to continuously reconstruct expectations through communications – with the very real possibility of misunderstanding and rejection of what is communicated).

This is a crucial point that those working with networks in the HST framework do not pay attention to. The reflexive communication clarifying and certifying the inclusion/exclusion of someone or some organization in certain communications is crucial (although still contingent) to define who is part or not of the network. If it is admitted that the organizations and individuals in a network do not take for granted inclusion or exclusion from the networks they participate in, the reflexive processes are needed to confirm the pertinence of the addressees (the members of the network) and further assure the continuity of the communication as relevant for the network. The network can only be established if such an arrangement for confirmation is used, which implies reflexive communication, i.e. communications about past communications in view of future communications. To represent such communication as a tie in a network, it is necessary to distinguish many types, strength of ties and those nodes that are connected by them. The current conceptualization of ties and nodes does not account for such distinctions, qualities, modes of operation and complexities.

In the same critical perspective, the metrics used to describe and portray networks with the respective quantitative descriptors (such as centrality and density of network nodes, for instance) do not capture any recursive communication process. Even the reciprocity indicator does not address this aspect. To observe the recursive nature of communication, the observer needs to follow sequences of communications over time. The social network analysis tool does not embrace diachronic orientation; it instead relies mostly on cross-sectional, synchronic and transversal cuts. Luhmann (2017b) mentions the role of reciprocity in establishing structural coupling between organizations, creating relations based on expectations and their fulfilment over time. However, reciprocity is a fragile link, he reminds us, as the autopoiesis each participant pursues cannot fully rely on it.

In addition to these critical views, if a system is considered to be self-organizing, and therefore necessarily able to carry out self-observations, the network can be observed by the system itself, which could therefore change it (or not). The sentence above may be interpreted as a metaphorical expression of the capacity of the system to decide. Luhmann's theory extensively explains how systems decide through the connectivity and recursive nature of communications, which reflect on communicated meanings (by communicating about communication and confirming or not previous communications), and communicating selections to keep or change the communicated topics. This means that a decision can be communicatively taken inside a system to affect the network that the system is participating in or sustaining. On the contrary, a network cannot make decisions. A network itself does not have the capability of self-reflection and self-adjustments; this has to be done through the individual, operationally closed system's communications. The theory of networks does not foresee or address such complex self-referential possibilities, carried out by the individual systems/organizations. A network that involves different organizations cannot self-refer as a unit. In contrast, the organizations can do that, and assess their own roles and behaviours in the network, but the network does not have such capacity.

Additionally, while boundaries and the correlated operational closure are key concepts for understanding systems and systems operations, networks implies "dissolution of organizational boundaries", ignoring the essential role that defining membership and separation between members and non-members is vital for an organization's reproduction and survival.

The proponents and users of network analysis as a tool for health systems thinking do not account for these limitations. The implied vision of a system established as networks and therefore to be analysed with the proposed tools, cannot explain much and cannot be used for understanding health systems more comprehensively. It is necessary to acknowledge that there are two different paradigms, one constituted by nodes and ties making up networks, and the other by autopoietic self-referred communication-based systems.

To be sure, Luhmann makes reference to networks in several of his works. Networks may appear as the connection of elements internal to the system, communicating to each other according to channels and programmes the system adopted. Besides that, he acknowledges that systems can enter into structural coupling with each other and these stable relations can configure networks; however, these networks do not perform autopoiesis on their own; instead, the systems and organizations making the networks indeed carry out their autopoiesis individually and that is what gives life to the network (not the opposite). This leads to the conclusion that, because of networks' subordination to the autopoiesis of the organizations/systems establishing them, networks are unstable and vulnerable.

In short, from the Social System Theory perspective, networks come into existence through the decisions taken by participant organizations/members. Even if the networks thus established can have influence over the decisions the organizations may take once the networks are in place, the networks remain reliant on the decisions taken by the organizations, which value their self-reproduction with higher priority over the maintenance of any agreed – implicitly or explicitly – network arrangement.

A still controversial conclusion could be that although systems operate with and within networks, and there are links and ties an external observer may consider characteristic of specific networks, any system has more elements and relations than the concept of the network can describe. The life of a function system does not essentially rely on any particular network or particular components of any network.

The life of the system relies on the communications that happen inside it, whether these communications can be understood within a given network or not. Many patients meet their doctors many times a day. They always communicate, but they often do not belong to the same networks. They may communicate once in their lifetime and never see each other again. This is often the case. It would require stretching the idea of a network too far to include such specific encounters that do not recur. The point is that not all that concerns meaningful communications is relevant for networks, but they are, by definition, part of the system. The communications between doctors and patients certainly happen in their millions every day and are relevant for the health systems.

Furthermore, the concept of the network does not account for individual systems' operations, although they may use some network to perform them. For instance, communication may (not necessarily) go through established networks, but the network itself does not account for the linkages, recursive processes, successes or failures of meaning-carrying communications. An existing network may indicate pathways for some communications between organizations, but success or failure cannot be foreseen from the network structure, although many empirical works have tried to demonstrate this and ended up with contradictory conclusions; for instance, a denser network structure may facilitate the rapid spread of information or, by the same token, be an obstacle to introduction of new information (Blanchet and Shearer 2017).

The cause of the mismatch between the expectations of what the theory of networks is supposed to gain in predictive power and what it actually delivers is a consequence of a lack of consideration of the contingency of links and nodes, and changes. Network ties and nodes are contingent, meaning they are neither necessary nor impossible, and can be different. Admitting their contingence implies the acceptance that they can change very often; they are not "written in stone". The circumstances that make them meaningful are also changeable. In short, the network is always a "work in progress", with "plans and designs" being defined and constantly modified. The illusion of fixity and permanence that cross-sectional studies may grant immunizes against the discomfort of recognizing many contingencies and complexities, but, on the other hand depletes the capacity to understand the system, as well as making predictions.

Putting it differently, it seems that network analysis makes efforts to reduce complexity and by doing so can end up with too simplistic a view of the observed phenomena. In the words of John Law:

> the notion of the network is itself a form – or perhaps a family of forms – of spatiality: that it imposes strong restrictions on the conditions of topological possibility. And that, accordingly, it tends to limit and homogenize the character of links, the character of invariant connection, the character of possible relations, and so the character of possible entities. (Law and Hassard 2005, p. 7)

In other words, nodes and links are far more diverse than the standardized "homogenized" elements that network analysis assumes; the reality is more complex than presumed.

To conclude, what has been said is not an attempt to entirely disqualify network analysis as a possible useful tool. The tool can indeed be useful for understanding particular operations of a health system. What it does not provide though is an understanding of what a health system is. Researchers may be able to find countless networks inside health systems and health organizations; it just depends on the topic in which the researcher is particularly interested. The researcher can look at the system, and find there may be such and such networks operating in it or linking the system to other systems or linking different organizations. But we need to understand that a collection of diverse networks or network possibilities does not make a system. The researcher will need to differentiate the internal networks, which have specific relevance for the system self-reference and self-organization, and external ones that are established for reasons guiding the system in its approaches to its environment. But, as said, the system has a "nature", so to speak, that engulfs all its component networks. It is the system that defines, creates, maintains, reproduces and terminates its networks, not the other way round. Systems pursue their autopoiesis while networks don't. As discussed by Bommes and Tack (2006), comparing organizations (as a type of autopoietic system) and networks, organizations are constituted by decisions while networks are made by relations of reciprocity, therefore, in their words: "the dynamics of organizational decisions tend to destroy the subtle structures of reciprocity" of networks (Bommes and Tack 2006, p. 301).

Summary of key concerns:

1. The tautology by which nodes are made by ties, and ties by nodes, and nodes and ties make up the structure of the network that determines the ties and the nodes of the network creates a recurrence that needs to be stopped at some point. However, the circularity does not incorporate theoretical elements that could break the tautology, for instance when the structure determines the behaviour instead of being determined by the behaviour of the nodes and ties.
2. The weakness of the SNA in addressing changes in time is well acknowledged by those working with this tool. There have been attempts to solve this problem with more sophisticated software capable of handling the data collected from the same network at different moments in time. The

difficulty is that the explanation of the changes will always be sought outside the frame of the SNA itself, because the SNA theory does not identify dynamic factors to explain how a network may develop in one direction instead of another.

3. SNA does not incorporate contingencies. Social systems have contingencies in all their dimensions.
4. A network is not a system; it does not have the structure of a system. It only describes some of the features and relations that may exist inside a system and between the system and its environment.
5. SNA does not account for the specificities of communications. It reifies ties as if once they are said to exist they become an essential part of reality. Therefore, it does not account for the fact that both nodes and ties are contingent and neither necessary nor impossible.
6. An important aspect of communication that is not incorporated into the SNA models is the recursive nature of communication (by which communication can be used to clarify, confirm, change, adjust, and make expectations etc. about previous and future communications). This functionality is of high importance for keeping the autopoiesis of any social system based on communication. It is not only relevant to know that A shared information Y with B, but also that B let A know that he understood what A had said and A checked whether that understanding was indeed correct or needed corrections. The back and forth of communication processes are vital for system survival, but SNA does not pay attention to this. A network tie is hurriedly assumed to be perfectly functional at the point the researcher identifies it.
7. The position of the observer is not a theme or point of concern in SNA. The fact that the observer is outside the network or belongs to it as a node does not seem to be relevant for SNA. On the contrary, Social Systems Theory highlights the need to be aware of the observer's position.
8. Finally, by radically removing complexities and narrowing down the system to homogenized and standardized nodes and ties, the network analysis unavoidably ends up with too simplistic and particularistic a narrative of the system it intends to describe.

5.3 Boundary critique

In spite of the explanations given by the proponents of the boundary critique (BC) technique (Reynolds and Wilding 2017), clarifying that it is not a research method but a reflective approach to methodological design, the BC can be examined for what it is proposed to do, i.e. indicate how to make boundary judgements. They say: "making boundaries judgements constitutes the core of systems thinking. Wherever the term 'system' is used ... there are implicit or explicit boundaries invoked" (Reynolds and Wilding 2017, p. 39).

The authors do not make an explicit definition of what boundaries are or what they separate. They say that: "boundaries mark out the map (systems of interest) from the territory (messy or 'wicked' situations of interest)" (Reynolds and Wilding 2017, p. 39), but this does not help much to identify what is being separated from what by whatever boundary one is talking about. The separation of "map" and "territory" and how boundaries are drawn between them is as confusing as the separation of "interests" and "situations of interest" and the connection between these two distinctions.

A second attempt, though still not a fully articulated definition, appears on page 40, referring to a triangle proposed by Ulrich (1996, as referenced by the authors), using notions of value judgements, fact judgements and boundary judgements. Although calling attention to the role of the observer in figuring out the relevance of these judgements, how a system will become visible from those judgments remains obscure. For an observer equipped with Social Systems Theory concepts, facts, values and boundaries become relevant as they enter the communications inside the system, when the system self-referentially communicates about those matters (more on this later)

The authors also propose a critical system heuristics (CSH) – a guiding enquiry tool comprising 12 questions for developing a model of the system being studied. The 12 questions are entries in a 4 x 3 matrix, where the 4 rows represent sources of influence (in their words: motivation, control, knowledge and legitimacy), and the 3 columns represent stake-holding references for making boundary judgements (to say: stakeholders, stakes and stake-holding issues).

The proposed tool looks like a rather complicated arrangement, as it is difficult to figure out what sort of system boundaries will then be drafted combining the answers to the 12 questions in a meaningful identification of a system's limits (distinguishing the system from whatever might be on the other side). Instead, the outlook of the elements of the matrix resembles a list of points for an exploratory assessment intended to identify the relevant issues a researcher should take into account while trying to understand a specific system. However, there is no definition of systems as such in the approach. Neither the concept of system nor of the boundaries and the respective attribution of what is separated from what become clearer with the proposed enquiry.

We can contrast this impressionistic approach to boundaries with Luhmann's precise notion of systems' boundaries. According to Luhmann: "Biological systems distinguish themselves from their environment by means of spatial material boundaries Psychic and social systems are not material in the same sense. Their material condition are part of their environment but do not enter into the autopoieses of their specific medium, which is meaning" (introduction by Peter Gilgen on page xv of *Introduction to Systems Theory* by Luhamnn 2013). "The boundaries of social and psychic systems are therefore not material artefacts but two-sided forms, which is to say, distinctions." In other words, the boundaries are constructed at the level of meanings, whereby the system recognizes, through distinctions, the meanings that are relevant for it, and discards the rest.

In the chapter on "Operational Closure" in the same book, Luhmann says:

The distinction between system and environment is produced by the system itself. This does not exclude the possibility that a different observer observes this distinction, which is to say, observes that a system exists in an environment. From the viewpoint of the thesis of operational closure, the important issue consists in the fact that the system draws its own boundaries by means of its own operations, that it thereby distinguishes itself from its environment, and that only then and in this manner can it be observed as a system. (Luhmann 2013, p. 63)

This theoretical perspective defines precisely what boundaries are. Boundaries are thus drawn by the system in operations distinguishing itself from its environment, and thus establishing itself as a system. It is important to keep in mind that when Luhmann speaks of operations, he is talking about communications.

The authors of the chapter describe an example where their approach to boundaries is applied. The case study is a partnership between several institutions in the context of a comprehensive policy for urban, social and health services development.

Had the authors' approach been informed by Luhmann's explanations about the role of boundaries and how they are constituted in correspondence to the systems/environment distinction, they could have reached different conclusions. They perhaps would have recognized that, before entering a partnership, each organization involved has already constructed its boundaries, distinguishing itself from its environment in ways fundamental to its existence and reproduction. All other organizations, whether in the same partnership or not, belong to the environment not to the organization (as a system).

They would then see that the question of boundaries in a partnership has to be addressed from the point of view of each organization's self-definitions, vital for their self-identity and internal operations. Coupling with other institutions may or may not be of interest vis-à-vis the organization's self-references. Their own boundaries, as self-defined, are more important for the preservation and continuity of their operations than any partnership per se; no matter how strong the political pull to bring institutions together, combining them into a single partnership unit.

A partnership therefore never supersedes the autopoietic drive of each individual organization participating in it. Partnership is only meaningful as long it is coherent with the autopoiesis of the organizations taking part in it. This is the logical conclusion the Social System Theory could suggest in relation to boundaries and partnerships. The theory thus does some work for the researcher. If a theory is not well designed or not made explicit in the investigation process, the researchers will struggle with the fluidity of aspects that are always changing and can only be observed contingently.

According to the proponents of the critical system heuristics, boundaries should be pointed at according to 12 possible combinations of sources of influence and the stakes, stakeholders and stake-holding. It looks rather a patchy network of several bits and pieces of possible relations between elements in a mosaic, lacking a sense of unit or integration. The impression is of a collage without perspective, as if the observer tries to apprehend a system addressing many of its details in a vain attempt to grasp the whole, ending up with the suspicion that there are many boundaries and they can be constructed in many ways.

No system would operate as such if it had to address its boundaries following so complex an approach. It would collapse. The point is that systems need to clearly define their boundaries in simple terms to prevent being overwhelmed by the complexities of the environment. They need to know and they do know where they set the boundaries. If boundaries are defined as the line that separates communications that are meaningful from those with no meaning for the operations of the system, things become a lot clearer and more precise.

We are certainly not talking about spatial boundaries, and the spatial metaphor (of maps and territory) does not help much in understanding a system's boundaries. However, any system made up of communications can know which communication should be considered relevant and which should be discarded or ignored altogether. The differentiation of many systems in the same society is achieved by this process, through which each system individually separates what is from what isn't relevant for it.

Where doubts might be raised, answers can be found within the system itself. If the observer is an operator inside the system, using the communication codes of the system to generate, receive and reply to legitimate communications, they will know what to do, how far they can go and where the communication should stop. A health professional in a hospital perfectly distinguishes what are the matters of health/sickness they should be concerned about. Even if the employed semantics and meanings go through transformations and changes, the processes will run with full continuous cross-checking and guarantees that whatever is internally communicated is relevant and therefore should (or should not) be part of the system. Everything else belongs to the environment – belongs to the other side of the boundary. That is a precise way of defining boundaries.

Surely there are communications about issues classifiable as related to "values", "power", "knowledge" and "morals", the four "sources of influence" of the framework, and these communications may involve "stakeholders", "stakes" and "stake-holding issues", as established in the CSH. However, the system itself elects mechanisms to live with such internal complexities. For its autopoiesis, the system relies on codes and programmes that can select the topics according to criteria of relevance, as far as the topics and themes are indeed of matters the system needs to communicate about.

In line with the Social System Theory, for the constitution of a partnership between organizations, the point of departure would be the acknowledgement by all partners that each corresponds to a fully established system, i.e. they are equally entities with the required attributes to operate as a system. This means that all are already aware that their organizations have their boundaries, have their on-going operations and keep the daily flows of communications by which they communicate as they need, in line with their core purpose and reproduction aims.

So, no one is naive. In being a member of an organization, one is committed to it; the commitment is inherent to membership. Without that clear-cut definition of who is a member of which organization, neither the organizations nor the partnership would survive the first meeting. Once the recognizance and acceptance of this basic constitutive characteristic of each partner is reached, then the progress can be measured in terms of designing and proposing "coupling" mechanisms that are of interest for all.

The partners will be constructing together the coupling details, by which their boundaries are preserved. At the same time, room for joint initiatives is created, fully recognizing and respecting the boundaries that constitute each partner. Even if they proceed with as much openness as they may choose, an external observer may not grasp the boundaries being preserved, but each organization will clearly distinguish and observe what concerns it.

Each organization will observe its partners, and as observer it will choose the distinctions to employ. The joint effort may consist in aligning the distinctions so that every partner will be able to assess the others in the same terms as each is assessed, including self-assessment, in the context of the partnership.

But the perspectives can never be fully aligned because the observers have diverse perspectives of observations, and the issues of their own organizations will have prevalent weight in the considerations for making observations.

Nevertheless, partnerships and coupling are possible, as long as the boundaries are acknowledged clearly. For instance, each one's budget is each one's matter and cannot be shared or submitted to decisions external to the organization itself. This is just an example that partnership will have its limits when the inner life of a partner cannot be invaded by the attention or interest of the others. These sketched points seem to be a more promising approach to system boundaries.

5.4 Process mapping

Process mapping (Muñoz and de Savigny 2017) considers activities that depart from decision nodes in mutually exclusive directions. A decision node indicates that the subsequent activity will be either of two options. This representation of decisions portrays formalized steps of idealized sequences, which although helpful in providing a visual idea or mental map of how the process should evolve, exclude a number of important aspects.

This tool is not based in any theory of systems and could therefore be employed as a managerial tool for dealing with specific types of organizational problems involving flows of information. There is nothing specifically related to systems in it. It can be considered a redressing of tools such as "flow charts" or O&M (organization and methods) developed in the 1950s and 1960s to make clear diagrammatic representations and descriptions of organizations' activities, emphasizing the connection between the steps and the coherence of sequencing to achieve the desired results. The tool can be compared with the step-by-step computer programming languages widely available in the 1960s.

Obviously the intention in drawing such schematic maps is reduction of the complexities it permits, or, in other words, the "taming" of complex realities into a selected arrangement of links and steps that wipe out the discomfort of noises and interference. However, if one considers what has thus been removed – if for instance one has Luhmann's theory in mind and asks: "Where are the communications?" – the tool can be assessed in a different light.

According to Luhmann, organizations are social systems built by communications. In fact, at each step of any mapped process, one can expect that there should be communications between those involved, at both the sending and receiving ends of any step in the process. Communications are crucial for the actual occurrence of the expected activities. If one side does not understand the communications (or rejects them), it is unlikely that the activity will unfold as it has been mapped out.

The framework ignores communication and the inherent double contingency, taking for granted that the parties involved at each step of the processes know precisely what actions are expected from them, and will act accordingly because the mapped process implies clear rationales for everyone involved. Often, this is not the case. The individuals involved may not perform as expected for many different reasons.

The civil registration and vital statistics (CRVS) example presented in Muñoz and de Savigny chapter is valuable in that sense; families do not accept or do not care about (do not have the need or incentive for) doing what is expected from them in terms of taking the medical notification of death to the District Registration Office. They may be clearly told (or not clearly or not at all) to do that; they may have understood (or not) what they have been told, but they may have forgotten or perhaps refused to follow the instruction; they may not communicate any of these possible "unexpected" alternatives to the officers involved, and the officers may never know what has happened next and why.

Because communication is so crucial it must be included in the analytical framework. If there is interest in making sense of processes, the occurrences and successes of communications have to be assessed. The recursive nature of communication, by which it can repeatedly go back and forth to ensure understanding and possible compliance, is one of the characteristics of communication that needs to be taken into account. For purposes of guarantee, understanding can be assumed to be an unlikely outcome of communications.

From Luhmann's theory, one may also consider the "operational closure" of the system. Not all elements in a process involving clients or external players or stakeholders can be considered as part of the system. If they are not identified members of the system/organization, with their respective roles and sets of expectations about their behaviour, the coupling with the system is loose. They may or may not fulfil the expectations because the consequences for complying (or not) may not be relevant, as opposed to a member of the system to that effect.

Analysed from this perspective, process mapping should give different weights for different participants in the process. In a continuum from those for whom certain expectations are considered highly relevant, to the other extreme, of those who are completely indifferent, or even against the expectations, the variation can have a crucial effect on the outputs of a process.

Process mapping is a planning tool. As mentioned above, computer languages, available since the late 1950s (like Fortran from 1957 and COBOL from 1959), used diagrams that are very similar to those proposed for process mapping. The step-by-step sequencing of operations, with the conditional decisions in between, orienting the direction of the flow of logical decisions and calculations, is suitable for computer programs where external interferences are 100 % under control – a situation that cannot be likened to the processes inside an organization or between organizations and elements in their environment.

These social processes have to rely on many contingencies that cannot be taken for granted. Contingencies means that things can be different, and communication involves double contingencies because both sender and recipient of the messages can always make different selections of what they communicate about. One can either ignore the contingencies, running the risk that things will be different from the expectations, or try to incorporate them in the uncertainties, to critically consider as inherent uncertainties any that cannot easily be accommodated within the precise logic of process mapping.

Additionally, an organizational process is a relation between acts and things that surely has been established by a decision taken at some point in the life of the organization. Such a decision organizes the "world" and becomes, in Luhmann's terms, a "decision premise" for subsequent related decisions. Whether the decision is of an operational or strategic nature, or, in other words, a decision intended to keep activities in line with adopted processes or a decision to introduce new processes, the options are picked considering what had been previously decided.

In any case, a process is not unalterable. It is contingent (can be different). Because of that, processes rely on the preservation of the expectations that created them in the first place; however, these expectations may not be maintained in the implementation of the processes. These uncertainties are not considered when mapping processes.

Those who initiate the processes and those who correspondingly follow the prescribed subsequent steps all have expectations in relation to what will come to them and what they will deliver next. They also acknowledge that the ones above or below any given point in the processes also have expectations. Several communications (by oral utterances, or paperwork, or electronic messages, etc.) are expected to follow the chains of expectations, up or downwards from any given point.

However, communications are contingent and often need confirmation, or back and forth to assure the correctness of the understanding and adequacy of the subsequent step.

These peculiarities of communications are not addressed in process mapping. Process mapping gives the illusion that once a process reaches a decision node it can only go in one of the predefined directions, while in the reality of communicative interactions such characterization of nodes is often not the case. The communication may go backwards for clarifications, corrections, or because of errors of interpretation and misunderstanding along the line. Processes do not accommodate well such reversal of directions; as models, processes reflect the irreversibility of time, always moving ahead, even with the artifice of incorporating feedback loops that may move the process back to a previous step. In fact, a feedback loop is still "a process moving forward", in contrast with a communication that goes backwards because a decision was not made or to request clarification or additional instructions.

The existence of mental representation of processes does not guarantee their correct implementation, their stability and immunization against misunderstandings at every single moment. Processes change by design or by practice (or lack of it), and mapping them only provides very limited assurance of their reliability or even correspondence to reality.

If processes are mapped as actions or activities, they lose the crucial connective "glue" of communication, which assures that those involved in a process actually share the same understanding of what is being communicated and therefore act as expected. Communication has inherent features that actions do not have. Without proper communication, the processes have a high chance of breaking down. As opposed to communication, action does not inherently require recurrent confirmation or subsequent interlacing; Luhmann is eloquent in affirming communication as the only pre-eminently social action, as it can only happen with the concurrence of at least two individuals and requires understanding (including misunderstanding) to be accomplished, while any other type of action may end in itself without producing interlacements. In his words: "'Action' first of all refers to an individual human being and not to a process that links different human beings" (Luhmann 2013, p. 183).

The lack of adequate theoretical framework has undermined the construction, application and self-critique of the utilization of this tool. The study of prescribed or practised flows of information is obviously useful for representing, planning and improving existing routines. However, such an undertaking is far from enough to capture crucial aspects of the life of the system.

We make next a final comment on this tool, reflecting on how Social System Theory could approach civil registration and vital statistics problems, putting the issue in a new light. We can consider that families can be classified as systems as they have the characteristics of the organization type of system as described by Luhmann – which is to say, they are constituted based on membership and they have internal decision-making communicative operations in which only members can participate. These are the two central features of organizations as social systems: membership with decision-making prerogatives.

As systems, families can enter into structural coupling with other systems, such as with the governmental organizations providing social benefits (pensions, financial support, etc.), educational services (providing scholarships, school fees exemptions, etc.), health services (providing user-fee exemptions, specific healthcare support, etc.), judicial decisions (for inheritance of assets, etc.). The families need to produce death certificates to gain access to some of these benefits, according to countries' legislation.

The families will see and value the relevance of having a death certificate when they need to negotiate their way through the respective bureaucracies. The certificates become a fundamental piece in the communicative exchanges between the families and the institutions. Once the established legal and institutional structure of the country makes a death certificate an essential element for decision-making, the families, reflecting this characteristic of their environment, incorporate the death certificate as a theme in their internal communications. Once that is achieved, the effects are clearly felt in the respective bureaucratic apparatus. Otherwise, the families might just carry on without registering the deaths of their members, as they will not see any advantage in having to go through the ordeal, spending time and money dealing with institutions.

In conclusion, a systems approach to the problem of CRVS will, first of all, need to recognize the systems and organizations involved and, considering their functionalities, assess the linkages between them. The exclusive focus on process details may hinder the acknowledgement of the larger picture where the systemic aspects effectively play the key roles.

5.5 Causal loop diagram

Usually presented as diagrams and therefore known as causal loop diagrams (CLD), this tool has been incorporated into the HST literature with the explicit acceptance that health systems are governed by and have causal loops embedded in them (Tomaia-Cotsel et al. 2017). In its simplest version, a causal loop may consist of a recurring linear cause–effect link. It can also describe a binary decision according to a defined threshold (thermostat model, switching on/off a loop according to measurements of temperature). Advanced diagrams may include more complex combinations of variables and causal links and scales. Nevertheless, the "governed by" assertion needs to be assessed critically.

The chapter written by Tomaia-Cotsel et al.[2] in fact refers to representations of "mental maps" of assumed causal relationships between variables relevant for addressing a given problem, where loops may be presumed. Such mapping exercises may obtain large sets of variables to be subsequently reduced to a few that can reveal a consistent and simplified "one cause, one effect" relationship with possible recurrences. A loop, representing a positive or negative effect over key causes may then be proposed to explain the problem and indicate solutions. Obviously this is an observation technique deployed by the interested researchers. The researcher can be located inside the system but can also be an external observer with academic interests. The attempt to reduce complexity is a tenet of the tool.

---

2   Tomaia-Cotsel, A. et al. (2017) – *Causal loop diagrams: a tool for visualizing emergent system behaviour*, chapter 6 in in Applied Systems Thinking for Health Systems Research, a methodological handbook edited by De Savigny, D., Blanchet, K. and Adam, T.

If one accepts the understanding of systems as capable of self-reference, however, with continuous observation of their own operations and capacity to introduce changes in correspondence to the results of the observations, causal loops can hardly explain the dynamics driving a system. Even if loops actually exist in some instances, they cannot govern the system. This is the point we try to explain in this section, based on the Social System Theory.

In cybernetic terms, social systems are not *trivial machines* processing inputs and throwing outputs in a predetermined fashion, until they run out of inputs or processing capacity. Essentially, as mechanisms of *trivial machines*, feedback loops operate in a "blind mode", repeating themselves until they are somehow interrupted. In this sense, closed loops are artificial and cannot be used for predicting the behaviour of real social systems. To understand social systems, in relation to the external sources contributing with inputs, it is necessary to add decision-making dynamics such as coordination and supervision, to keep the loops operating, adjusting or switching them off if required.

An attempt to absorb the role of loops into the understanding of systems should try to reconcile the idea of loops with the notion that systems have a self-reference drive to perform self-preservation and self-maintenance (autopoiesis), for which they set in motion their self-organizing capabilities. In line with Social Systems Theory, a system needs to maintain its distinction from its environment, and by its own means preserve its distinctive internal operations. The system chooses the criteria it uses both to select what it considers of interest in the environment, and to select the internal elements and processes as it sees fit.

These self-management functions are incompatible with "governed by" automatic causal and deterministic "trivial machine"-like loops. Self-management requires continuous reflections on the status of the system and its operations. To be sure, a system can make mistakes, which may even lead to its destruction; one of those potentially destructive dynamics is exactly the continuous operation of a loop that depletes the system of its resources.

In such cases, unconstrained causal loops with negative effects can lead a system to collapse, unless the consequences they generate are compensated somehow by the intake of resources, or the loop is properly managed, meaning it is adjusted as necessary or even switched off, as mentioned above.

A causal loop may have some determinant factors beyond the system's control; however, the self-reproduction of the system ensures that it can select the elements and the relevance of their determinations, particularly when they become matters of survival for the system. Systems face causal links between variables, but are not entirely dominated by them.

Furthermore, there is no way of assuring the functionality of a system that will be set with feedback loops controlled by other feedback loops controlled by another set of loops, and so on, in an endless chain of ever-increasing complexity. Such a system will be extremely vulnerable in consequence of its very complexity, curtailing its possibility of recognizing and adjusting itself to unexpected changes in its (internal or external) environment.

In a system's life, there are decisions, dilemmas and paradoxes that cannot be described in causal loop terms. The semantics of the dilemmas, tautologies and paradoxes have to be processed, solved and decided upon by "machines" that are, in the first place, *non-trivial*, or in other words are not "governed" by feedback loops.

Another feature of causal loops that deserves consideration is related to the fact that causal loops involving recognition of variables, selection or information and decisions require communications within the system. Indeed causal loops may be useful in stable and well-defined cycles, such as replenishment of drugs, avoiding stock-outs of critical medicines. However, the loops are operated by communications and they are subject to the double contingencies of expectations and selections at both communicating ends.

Communications are very different from and cannot be likened to models like electric, electronic or mechanical switches in control devices such as thermostats or airplane stabilizers. Even in a simple causal loop set in motion, for instance, to keep drugs stocks at the required level in a health facility, the unavoidable reliance on communications makes the loop vulnerable to all sorts of communication contingencies. The CLD tool does not account for that. Health system staff both on the side of requesting/receiving the drug replenishments and on the side of providing/dispatching them may face disruptions and adversities hampering their communications. It can be expected that in some contexts the drug supply mechanisms are more likely to be disrupted by countless factors than to operate regularly as designed.

As a last reflection, organizations constantly assess the internal and external environment of their operations and identify causal links (whether locked in loops or not) and especially the vulnerabilities and the risks involved for the operation of the enterprise. The techniques for doing so have been developed since management started to claim its scientific status. Enterprises all over the world have been seriously interested in identifying organizational models and possible cause-effect relations associated with the models.

The issues at stake have always been the achievement of efficiency and growth as well as development of distinct identity traits in competitive environments. Certainly the inventory of possible causal relations as well as interfering factors is and has always been of vital importance for any enterprise, whatever its nature. Organizations deploy a substantive portion of their observational efforts and create specific departments for that purpose. But, in this pursuit, efforts fixed on finding causal loops may hamper the self-referencing drive of the system rather than providing a helpful tool.

To be clear, the CLD is helpful as an auxiliary tool to model behaviours of variables of interest in a number of diverse scientific and management endeavours. The exercise to map out the variables of relevance and the relations between them is undoubtedly part of the techniques the systems can deploy in their efforts to internally represent the environment as well as making self-descriptions.

The system may identify loops that need to be observed and managed, as well as identifying the full range of other relevant variables outside the loops and, more importantly, having contingent decision influences over the inferred relations between variables. All selections a system makes are contingent, i.e. can be different; therefore causality can be fragile and explanations in traditional *trivial machines* terms are not very useful. In that regard, CLDs are very weak tools for the analysis of systems.

In short, causal loops do not reconcile well with the notion of selections and contingencies. In contingency terms, relations between variables can be otherwise as different selections can be made (by the observers and by those communicating). Selections are not determined beforehand by definite causal factors that have power over how observations should be done. The distinctions used for making observations are the object of selection. Selections are deliberations the system makes and communicates about. In the realm of communications, the selections can always be different. This goes to the heart of the epistemology of social systems.

To conclude, we can mention as an example that a biologist may find many causal links and possibly some loops among the interactions between different species in a forest. However, the ecology of the forest is not an autopoietic system as Social Systems Theory defines it. The interplay among species is an example of causal links between variables where neither the links nor the variables (species in the forest) comprise a system. Causal links and loops can exist without being part of a system. Autopoietic systems can address and incorporate causal links according to their relevance for their autopoiesis. This is essentially the confusion CLD makes between models and systems. Models are representations of sets of variables and the interactions (including possible causal loops) between them. In contrast, systems are autopoietic self-referred units communicatively controlling their own reproduction. In this sense, CLD is a good technique for modelling and problem-solving, but not for systems analysis.

Chapter 6 – Health Systems Strengthening and Systems Theory

This chapter discusses the horizons Luhmann's theory opens for studying health systems strengthening (HSS). For Social Systems Theory, if an operationally closed self-referential autopoietic system can be strengthened, that has to be done by the system in correspondence with its essential prerogative of reproducing itself. Therefore the chapter explores the questions on how a system can become more capable of self-reproduction, or, in other words, how it can use self-assessment to "improving".

In fact, in Luhmann's texts we do not find references to system "strengthening". In his theory, a system either performs its autopoiesis or no longer exists. A system's competence to perform autopoiesis, i.e. to produce the means for its own reproduction, is all that is needed.[1] The strengthening of a system therefore is a matter of the system's handling through communications the complexities it observes in the environment and in itself, ensuring its self-reproduction.

The chapter extensively discusses this topic, starting with a debate on how HSS initiatives can be analysed from the Social Systems theoretical point of view, with a specific section dedicated to the topic of *resilience*. Furthermore, the chapter discusses the relations between political systems and health systems, and concludes with some reflections on complexity and systems strengthening.

---

1   As mentioned in previous chapters, Luhmann (2013) says social systems, like biological systems, rely on the environment as a source of energy and materials, but all information the system needs is produced internally. A system can observe the environment but not get information from it; the observations are translated into information inside the system.

6.1 Applying the theory – health systems strengthening

This section summarizes the conceptual characterization of systems from Luhmann's perspective, identifying the crucial elements for a discussion about strengthening health systems. The paragraphs below list what can have strengthening implications in a health system.

In Social Systems Theory terms, systems strengthening should be based on a number of functionalities related to improvements in the capacities of the system to perform its reproduction, i.e. to ensure the terms and conditions of *self-reproduction* with the system managing its own *complexities* as well as the complexities it deals with in its environment. For that, the system/organization: reassures its competence for *self-observation* and *decision-making*; assures continuous internal *communication* of information generated and validated by itself; guarantees the consistency of its *internal differentiation* in sub-systems; preserves its unit at the same time as *coupling* with other systems; and strives to achieve enhanced capability to internally communicate *more complex information*.

From this perspective, strengthening a health system is conceived differently from the prevalent view that treats health systems as if they were large corporations (public or private or mixed), to be approached with managerial optics, attentive to comprehensive coordinated improvements to the "building blocks" (WHO 2007). Instead, from a social system point of view, health systems cannot be likened to features of large enterprises or "production functions", combining human, material, financial, and managerial resources. Even in organizations, as a distinct type of system (based on decision-making and membership), their systemic autopoietic reproductive dynamic does not equate to "production functions" components. Furthermore, the health system as a whole, as a function system, does not operate as an organization, although it may have many organizations operating inside it.[2]

Ultimately, in Luhmann's perspective, only the system can strengthen itself. With this in mind, we list below the key concepts of the theory for assessing the strengthening of a system.

---

2   In this discussion, It is important to remember that function systems and organizations are two different types of autopoietic social systems, as explained in the initial chapters.

1. *Communication* – the preservation of the on-going connectivity of the communications in the system is fundamental, preserving memory, codes, channels and utterances (including specific syntax, mediums and programmes). Information and utterances are to be maintained at the level they can be selected and understood, connecting past and future communications across the parts of the system; Particularly, and most importantly, communications related to diagnostics and treatments, key communication themes constituting a health system. Communications that are too complex to be processed or too simple – and below the level the system can deal with – are likely to be ignored, without connecting to subsequent communicative operations. To be sure, any act in a health system is made possible and becomes meaningful due to the communications that came before it, go with it or follow from it. In short, a system can only be strengthened to the extent its communications allow and are part of the strengthening process.
2. *Observation of the environment* – the system must observe its environment and for that deploy the distinctions the system makes/adopts. Distinctions need to be internally preserved as part of the repertoire/memory/identity of the system. The system needs to internally communicate the observations and selections it makes, together with the distinctions deployed. It should internally preserve and reproduce the internal capacity to select and use distinctions, perform the respective observations and communicate them. The body of the patient is part of the environment where the system deploys its observational distinctions. The strengthening of a system requires preservation of the system's acquired observational competences and the acquisition of new ones.
3. *Self-observation* – a system capable of observing the environment is also able to observe its effects on the environment and how the system itself has produced those effects; therefore such a system has self-observation capabilities. This implies that the system observes its way of producing distinctions and observations, and observes how internally it interprets (generating information) what it observes in the environment. In cybernetic jargon, such systems are capable of carrying out second-order observations. Self-observation is for instance exerted in processes such as monitoring and evaluation programmes, by which the system assesses the communications involved and therefore its own implementations. A system's competences for self-observation must be included as possibilities for self-strengthening;

4. *Handling of complexity* – Observation is also observation of the limits of comprehensibility or, in other words, observation of the limits of complexity the system can handle in the environment as well as in itself. The system selects communications and communication themes it recognizes as pertinent in line with its capacity to respond. Excessive complexity is thus avoided. This complexity reduction strategy, though, does not eliminate complex operations the system is already able to perform. The strengthening of the system should imply both the preservation of the competences to address complexities that the system has already achieved, as well as expansion of these capacity to address more complex problems, without threatening the integrity of the system. The strengthening of a system should enable it to make the necessary distinctions in assessing the levels of complexities (internal and external) it is facing.
5. *Operational closure and decision-making* – A system's observations develop from the basic distinction between system and environment (the distinction that creates the system). This distinction establishes the limits within which the system recognizes itself, preserving itself as an open system, as far as observation of the environment is concerned, and as a closed system, in relation to the generation of information – in other words, the system is open for observing the environment, and at the same time closed in its processes of internally generating all information it uses. Only information internally generated can be used for systems communication. For a system based on decisions (organizations), decision-making is its exclusive prerogative; only decisions it makes itself are recognized as belonging to it and therefore considered valid. In this sense, the recognition, acceptance and incorporation of rulings coming from the political and the legal systems become possible by internal deliberative processes in correspondence with external norms. Strengthening a system therefore means improving its operational closure; the contrary will lead to the destruction of the system.
6. *Autopoiesis* – As mentioned several times before, a system either performs its autopoiesis or no longer exists. Communication is the base of social systems autopoiesis. The system has to generate, control and maintain the communications it recognizes as belonging to it; in doing that, it carries out its autopoiesis. Just as a reminder, autopoiesis is the reproduction of a system using the means it creates itself. A function system like health also communicates about the generation of the competences for and the validation of communications. By doing that, the system reproduces the

conditions to continue producing communications in a consistent manner. Strengthening a system should therefore mean the same as the system making itself able to continuing its autopoiesis.

7. *Differentiation* – What defines a system as such is the system/environment distinction. A system is identified as differentiated from its environment, including all the other systems in it. The differentiation of a system's domains comes with the system's prerogatives of applying its codes and programmes the way it decides. This creates self-reference (the system referring to itself) and its opposite, hetero-reference (the system referring to what is not it). Besides this differentiation, a system may also establish internal differentiations, by which it creates internal sub-systems and, by doing so, the system improves the handling of complexities. A system's internal differentiation may enhance operational competences and internally stabilize patterns of communications linking internally differentiated sub-systems. Internal differentiation therefore equips a system with operative sub-systems with specific purposes for handling specific aspects of its autopoiesis, releasing other parts of the system from the same concerns. This increases and simplifies the processes of selection and, crucially, acceptance of communications. An example may help to see this apparently difficult conceptualization. For instance, the works carried out by professional councils ensures that the professional standards of communications (and related actions) are monitored and maintained. The healthcare service delivery components do not need to do the normative work the professional councils do. As another example, the health system differentiates health specialities and in that way gains in capacity to address the complexities of each speciality field, selecting and orientating cases within the system in a way that reduces complexity; thus, the system also allows for enhanced complex performances in specific areas of the system, without overburdening the whole system with generalized complexities. For instance, these internal differentiations increase the probability of acceptance of communications taking place in the field of the specialities, which would otherwise overburden the system – a specialist in internal medicine and infectious diseases may not be able to talk about the effects of radiotherapy, for instance, but that would not constitute a problem for the system. In short, strengthening a system requires continuous handling of the differentiations by which the system distinguishes itself from other systems and its environment, and distinguishes and manages the internal sub-systems.

8. *Meaning and contingencies* – As communication-based systems, social systems operate on the basis of meaning and contingencies. Luhmann uses a formal definition of meaning as the unit of the actuality/potentiality distinction (the meaning of something is fixed in contrast to the sets of other potential meanings that it excludes). On the other hand, contingency means that things are neither necessary nor impossible, and therefore can be different. Meanings are contingent, therefore they can also be different; in consequence of that, a system needs to consistently preserve relevant meanings. This is achieved by memory and the connectivity between past, present and future communications, thus preserving the communicated meanings. A recursive process of communications within the system, clarifying and certifying that messages have been well understood (or not), also contributes to stabilize meanings. Stability relies on the possibility of going back retroactively to clarify whether the intended message was understood correctly. Strengthening a system therefore requires the enforcement of reliable mechanisms of recursively checking meanings as well as the correctness of the selections made for constituting and connecting them. On the other hand, contingencies need to be contained so that the idea that meanings could be different have to be avoided by resorting to mechanisms that reinforce the adopted meaning. For instance, resorting to the opinion of a high-qualified board of experts on the matter, conferring even an ethical dimension to the acceptance of experts' opinions. So, in its internal differentiation, a strengthened system elects mechanisms for reducing contingencies and preserving meanings. Strengthening a system implies therefore making the system increasingly able to manage its contingencies and preserve the meanings it works with.

Having said that, it should have become clear that from the Social System Theory perspective, system strengthening couldn't be judged in the same terms of managerial, governance or economic evaluations. The autopoiesis of a system cannot be thoroughly translated in terms of the indicators used for such evaluations. For instance, developing new expertise is not necessarily a matter of cost-effectiveness, efficiency, equity, good governance, profit-maximizing and so on; it is first of all a matter of acquiring competences in areas of communications with responses to new problems not yet incorporated into the system, and the system considers that it has to do something about.

The strengthening of a system does not mean the system has become more efficient, more effective, more equitable, less costly, more profitable, or has generated higher revenues or higher monetarily expressed benefits. All of that may happen and still the key aspect of the system is its self-reproduction by the means it produces itself. Similarly, successful though highly improbable biological organisms or species may develop features that are neither necessary nor efficient to survive in their environment, but they become reproductively possible and are carried forward. There is no necessary cost–benefit (or cost-effectiveness or efficacy, etc.) justification for keeping an autopoietic system alive. In the context of its autopoiesis, a system cannot plan to stop it – that would be a paradox; autopoiesis cannot incorporate a self-destruction aim. Any communicative operation that is incorporated and belongs to a system by definition concurs for a system's autopoiesis, therefore anything aiming at the destruction of the system is not recognized as belonging to the system and consequently is not incorporated in it. The environment may produce such things that constitute risks the system needs to avoid. And indeed the theory recognizes the possibility of the annihilation of a system. Preserving autopoiesis is therefore a paradoxical option between remaining alive or dying, which in other words means that these are not real options for any system, as in its autopoietic drive a system cannot decide to self-destroy. Autopoiesis does not foresee such a possibility.

This discussion is not immune from controversies. However, the message the theory brings is that the enhancement of the capacity of the system to reproduce itself by its own means is what strengthens the system, not its adaptation to external assessment indicators.

External guiding principles for system strengthening may become normative prescriptions for those applying HSS in a given country. The normative principles may carry ideological orientations, whereby the proponents set the parameters for judging a health system based on programmes developed elsewhere. For instance, principles orientating health sector management, prescribing standards and/or promoting views and values that became possible in other contexts. However, this may put in front of the country's system an ideological, normative and doctrinaire mirror in which the system may not see itself. It may see only a distorted image that does not account for the actual functionality of the system as seen from the perspective of those who are enabling its existence, participating in its reproduction, articulating resources, policy mandates and decisions. This illustrates potential frictions between external experts and those internally operating a system in a given country.

6.2 Applying the theory – resilience

Resilience is a term often used in discussions about health system strengthening. The term denotes a desirable quality of health systems by which the system is endowed with the capacity to endure adverse circumstances as well as "bounces back" from disruptive occurrences such as epidemic, wars, natural disasters, etc. Resilient systems are considered able to maintain or even improve their operations while facing important unpredictable challenges.

However, there are different views. The article "From Bouncing Back, to Nurturing Emergence: Reframing the Concept of Resilience in Health Systems Strengthening" by E. Barasa, K. Cloete and L. Gilson (2017) proposes to treat resilience in reference to complex adaptive systems (CAS), therefore countering the narrow understanding of resilience as "bouncing back" from shocks, expanding it to what the authors call "everyday resilience", independent from sudden distresses, incorporating CAS attributes of "absorptive, adaptive and transformative strategies".

This section argues that the debate about resilience would gain in clarity with the use of concepts from the Social Systems Theory. First, the term resilience, although currently conveying positive connotations of a characteristic that assures the continuity and the efforts of the system to improve, it does not eliminate negative connotations. Bad habits are also resilient. Old processes and practices are hard to change once they have proved to be effective as responses to what were at some point the on-going circumstances. The strong emphasis on the positive side of resilience, like many concepts commonly used in international health, such as "participation", "empowerment", "governance", "ownership", "change", "accountability", "political commitment" etc. does not eliminate negative possibilities that the same terms can refer to. The positive undertones with which these terms are used do not eliminate accounts of the same phenomenon without the normative positive meanings they are one-sidedly dressed up in.

Terms that suggest a possible black or white (good or bad) characterization in fact obfuscate the variations and nuances of the actual phenomena being observed. With widespread use, the terms may become loose and poorly specified or, at the other extreme, over-specified and thus with too narrow and rigorous a meaning to be useful. On the loose side, determination becomes non-specific, and therefore the terms are abandoned and replaced by newer also vague ones. Internal accountability, for instance, is also important in informal, corrupt, mafia-style criminal organizations. Because of that, the use of these terms needs additional qualifications, which narrow down and tailor them to the specific context they refer to. Therefore, in order to speak of resilience, it is necessary to be clear on what one is specifically talking about in each context.

The term "everyday resilience" muddles the indeterminacy a bit further. How to distinguish between the daily undertakings that effectively represent some sort of resilience, understood as continuity in the face of adversity, and undertakings that have difficulties and barriers that most undertakings usually have? Conditions are hardly perfect, whatever the level of requirements. Where can the line be drawn? How high should the uncertainties and threats become before the word resilience can be applied? Surely, health professionals who on a daily basis have to cross battlegrounds to reach their facilities demonstrate incontestable resilience. But these situations are very unusual. The proponents of the term seem to be referring to simple daily difficulties rather than dramatic extremes. But then, why not just call the professionals dedicated instead of resilient? Assisting women delivering their babies at night, using torchlights because the maternity hospital has not paid the electricity bill can be proof of dedication and willingness to work in difficult circumstances; is it necessary to call that resilience? Do health workers identify themselves with the adjective "resilient" or do they prefer to refer to themselves as dedicated, persevering, motivated and willing to do the job, without any connotation of endurance in face of adversity? This is a question in need of an empirical answer.

Moreover, the concept of autopoiesis in Social Systems Theory could be inadvertently likened to resilience, but that would not be correct. Autopoiesis means the system is reproducing itself by the means it creates itself. Besides that, a system that does not perform its autopoiesis ceases to exist. Autopoiesis has to go on whether the system is resilient or not, and the system has to reproduce itself by the means at its disposal, whether that implies resiliency or not.

The advantage of the concept of autopoiesis in relation to resilience is the fact that the system is always reproducing itself in whatever condition it is. If it stops, it dies. The concept calls attention to the mechanics of reproduction, and the role of communication in the process. The reproduction of the system is the reproduction of its communications. A system may carry on making the same mistakes and mistakenly communicate about them. Even though it will still reproduce itself and carry on with its autopoiesis. Therefore, what needs to be understood and analysed are the communications by which the system is reproducing itself. Resilience is not a satisfactory or helpful concept for studying these reproductive processes.

6.3 Applying the theory – the political and health systems

This section gives only a brief explanation of the political system's functions as seen from the Social Systems Theory point of view; this is just a summary of the conceptualization. Among the advanced topics covered in the Annex of the book, there is a section dedicated to relations between political and health systems. The text discusses power and the political system, complementing the theoretical views on the political system with notions about how power as a medium of communication works.

By following the previous discussions in this chapter, the understanding that the strengthening of the health system does not require the interference of the political system may have already come to mind when we discussed the prerogative of the health system to strengthen itself. We do need to take into account that the field of health policy is consolidated in the overarching umbrella of the public health subsystem. Health policy studies are predominantly concerned with the operations taking place in the political system, and how its decisions play a crucial role in shaping a health system. The studies scrutinize a plethora of potential players (many outside the health system) having a say in the public arena, affecting the final rulings. There is no way of denying the role of those players in shaping agendas and the outcome of the political debate. What we nevertheless still need to reflect on is the differentiation and the distinct closure by which the political system cannot be part of the internal communications of the health system. The coupling of the health and political systems is a very special subject in the application of the theory, particularly in relation to health systems strengthening.

In other words, the political system cannot participate in the communications inherent to the health system. The political system does not have the required competence to generate health communications and does not have the legitimacy to do so. Yes, as noted above, decisions taken by the political system can have high importance for the health system, but the operation of the health system, for instance communications about diagnostics and treatment of patients, is not a matter the political system can communicate about. There is a lot to unpack about these points, but as mentioned, these discussions are partially covered in the Annex, within the limits of the introductory scope of this book.

The political system

This brief presentation of Luhmann's description of the political system is intended to contrast the two differentiated functional systems: health and politics. The political system is of crucial relevance for health systems relying on public budgets as well as for any health system depending on political enactment of the legal regulations under which the health system operates. However, it is important to keep in mind that both are *operationally closed* systems pursuing their own autopoiesis independently.

Luhmann dedicated great deal of his efforts to describe the structure and functioning of the political systems. He wrote a number of books, book chapters and articles explaining how the system theory explains political systems. Again, in this book we cannot give the full breadth of his efforts, but the main lines of his thoughts are briefly explained:

1. Political systems have an internal differentiation and are composed of three partial systems: the political, the administrative and the public.
2. The life of a political system develops as couplings and de-couplings of these three partial systems.
3. Rather unusually, Luhmann's definitions of politics (as the executive exercise of political debate and pressure over areas of interest), the administration (combining the translation of politics into legal instruments and decisions as well as operational plans in correspondence to deliberations coming from the political sub-system), and the public (as not only public opinion but public voices that have political effects, influencing both the administrative and the political systems), has steered controversies. Luhmann's scheme does not neatly map out the usual separation between the three powers: executive, legislative and judicial;
4. As a function system, among all the other function systems, the political system does not occupy the centre of society.
5. The function of the political system is to produce *collectively binding decisions*.
6. The political system is mobilized to make decisions on issues concerning other function systems. When the political pressure finally rises to the point of forcing the system to act, the political system performs the processes of consultation, discussion, deliberation, and so on, and eventually

issues legal ordinances that are *collectively binding*. Collectively binding decisions is what justifies the existence of the political system.
7. The legitimacy of the political system is a never-ending concern for the system. It has to continuously confirm its mandate to produce collectively binding decisions that are accepted. Its legitimacy is constantly in need of confirmation to secure the acceptability of its decisions. The pursuit of legitimacy is what drives the recurrent coupling and de-coupling of the political system.
8. The political system is orientated by the binary code government/opposition (or government/governed).
9. Operational closure as seen in the other function systems is also characteristic of the political system, which communicates internally (among the three differentiated partial systems) in terms of its binary code, within the semantics that concerns and is related to the code.
10. The political system cannot perform operations inside any other function system. Despite the fact that the political system (particularly in welfare states) is constantly called to resolve the problems of other function systems (economy, health and education for instance) it has no capacity to do what is the prerogative of other function systems. That brings incessant stresses to the political system that, when possible, tries to avoid getting involved with other systems' problems.
11. The political system has a particular coupling with the legal system as the political decisions taken in the medium of power needs to be formed in the medium of law and then be incorporated into the operations of the legal system.
12. The legal system therefore realizes for the political system what it would not be able to achieve alone.

For those interested in knowing the political system better from the point of view of Luhmann, some of the key references are: Luhmann (1990), *Political Theory in the Welfare State*; Luhmann (2014), *Sociología Política*; King and Thornhill (2003), *Niklas Luhmann's Theory of Politics and Law*.

For our discussion, it is sufficient to note that the political system can have positive as well as negative effects when it comes to contributing to strengthening health systems. We are not talking here about the managerial/entrepreneurial or business dimensions of the health sector. We are talking about the health system as a communication-based autopoietic social system. Any influences that may reduce the capacity of the health system to perform its communication prerogatives affects it negatively and reduces its strength.

6.4 Applying the theory - complexity and health systems

As a last point, we address complexity. Complexity and complexity reduction are prominent concepts in Luhmann's theoretical architecture. The reader may have already noticed that complexity is a recurrent theme in this book. It is necessary to return to it often. The concept has been briefly explained in Chapter 2, and this brief section discusses complexity in health system in relation to system strengthening. How do health systems address complexities? And what are the effects of it in terms of system strengthening?

At the intersection of complexity and system science a range of questions arises on how systems respond to complexity in their environment and how the systems deal with their own self-observed complexities. First it is necessary to be clear that complexity and systems are two separate concepts. Complexity should be understood in reference to observational capacity. In this sense, complexity is not an ontological entity but rather a characterization deployed in observational processes, dependent on observational capacities to distinguish elements and relations between elements.

Complexity reduction and its opposite, complexity enhancement, can be observed and attributed to both sides of the system/environment distinction. In other words, complexity changes can be identified in the system as well as in the environment, within the limitations of the observer.

While the system itself has to become more complex in order to deal with the complexities it observes in the environment, the environment apparently becomes less complex. But that is only in the eyes of the system. In itself, the environment remains as complex as before. But it may also appear to become more complex, because the system starts to distinguish features in it that it was not able to see earlier.

That is simple to grasp if we consider as an example that medical equipment using magnetic resonance opened a perspective for scrutiny previously unseen. In that, we can say that both became more complex: the system, for being able to perform more sophisticate examinations, and the environment, as it now displays more diverse pictures of the examined tissues. In any case, complexity always refers to the capacity of the system to observe and the pictures it correspondently makes.

In previous chapter it was mentioned that a system does not have the "requisite variety" to represent the complexities of the environment on a one-to-one basis, meaning that the system cannot make inside itself entire copies of its environment. Systems are surely less complex than their environment. In consequence of that, health systems will need to constantly progress in their endeavour to know, identify and successfully prevent or treat diseases (new and old ones) appearing in the environment.

Diseases become more and more complex in correspondence to the system's competence to know and deploy increasingly complex ways to deal with them, looking more deeply into the details of the transformations the diseases bring about in bodies. Some authors, Bruno Latour among them, go a step further and say that new observation capacities create what then becomes observable – the microscopy created the bacteria. Social Systems Theory does not go that far. More precisely, the system strives to enhance its competence to collect new elements from the, so to speak, "limitless inventory" of known and unknown complexities of the environment.

By the same token, in enhancing its competences to investigate and treat diseases, the system also acquires complexities (multiple specialities are, for example, a good indicator of a system's complexity). A disease, the complexity of which is beyond the level of knowledge available in the system to identify and treat, will remain unrecognized, ignored or misrepresented.

In conclusion, strengthening is a matter of internal evaluation by which the system assesses whether its capacity to address the complexities it observes has increased. However, we can admit that there is another perspective: strengthening can be a judgement of the transformations the system has gone through; judgements made by external observers interested in seeing whether certain communicative competences have developed and can be found in the system. These are two different perspectives. Still, strengthening in both perspectives has to have expression in the communications capabilities of the system.

Chapter 7 – Health Organizations and Poly-contexturality

The analysis of health organizations such as hospitals, polyclinics, healthcare services complexes, clinical laboratories, etc. constitute a good test of the consistency of the Social Systems Theory. As organizations operate in several function systems simultaneously, as they have economic, political, educational, scientific, etc. interests, they are of high relevance for the theoretical architecture. Luhmann worked extensively on themes related to organizations. Organizations are one of the three types of social systems (*function systems*, *interactions* and *organizations*) and have differentiated functionality.

Chapter 1 presented the fundamental concepts of organizations as systems based on membership and decisions. For a general distinction, it can be said that while *function systems* work on the principle of inclusion, meaning all society members can in one way or another be included at some point in one or more function systems, organizations work on the principle of exclusion – that is, only members can be part of them, and participate in decision-making, while the rest of the society is excluded.

Decisions, decision premises, uncertainty absorption (see Chapter 1) are important concepts for understanding Luhmann's views on organization. Organizations have been also discussed in other chapters and sections of the book; this chapter, however, is exclusively dedicated to the "poly-contexturality" theme. This theme allows for a clear understanding of the functioning of complex organizations such as hospitals in the frame of the Social Systems Theory. In fact, Luhmann did not give prominence to the term "poly-contexturality"; it appeared in subsequent works based on the theory. However, it is indeed a useful conceptual tool for understanding health systems organizations.

A provider of health services a hospital is obviously in the health *function system*, but it is also in the economic system (as purchaser and seller of services and goods), in the education system (training doctors, nurses and others), in the legal system (dealing with court decisions on provision of healthcare services), in the political system (as politicians approve health budgets and investments), in the religious system (as religious rituals may be part of its daily life), in the science system (as a site for research on diagnostics and treatments), etc. The theoretical approach to organizations with such poly-contextures needs to reconcile key notions of Luhmann's theory, particularly the concept of *operational closure*.

The question therefore is how an organization such as a hospital, dealing with several *function systems*, preserves its *operational closure* and the *operational closure* of each *function system* involved. To answer this question, a number of aspects need to be considered.

Function systems differentiation defines socially recognizable distinct meaning domains. In the contemporary context of systems differentiation, any society member can have concurrent "addresses" in any *function system*. An individual can be a lawyer working in the legal system but can also be a teacher in the education system, a patient in the health system, a politician in the political system and so on. Having an address in a function system means having a socially recognizable location in that system, in roles the system recognizes (such as patient, doctor, nurse, etc.); that does not preclude having other addresses in other *function systems*. This configures the poly-contextural nature of contemporary society, with open possibilities for individuals' inclusion in different function systems simultaneously.

At organizations as social systems, the structural differentiation of society projects internal differentiations, with divisions dedicated to specific functions, with differentiated system/environment boundaries. For instance, the finance department of a hospital carries out communications in the economic system (buying and selling) in the environment of the organization. A modern organization therefore has multiple concerns, and this portrays the poly-contexture of health organizations, taking diverse orientations in diverse communication themes.[1]

Healthcare service delivery obviously is the core business of any health organization – its reason to exist as a socially recognized organization belonging to the health system. In organizations belonging to other function systems, the

---

1 For example, see Anna Henkel "Drugs in Modern Society: Analysing Poly-contextural Things under the Condition of Functional Differentiation", chapter 1 in Knudsen and Vogd (2015).

healthy/sick code cannot be deployed; the health system has the legitimate, exclusive prerogative to use it in diagnostic and treatment contexts.

However, other function systems are relevant for the operations of any organization, and the dealings with diverse function systems have to be done in complexity reducing ways. As treatments for illnesses remain the core business of hospitals, operations related to the other function systems must not overtax the central function of the health organization or distort its main purpose of identifying and treating diseases.

Internal differentiation is therefore needed, and achieved by developing internal distinct sub-units to deal with the specific observations required for communications with the other systems, without letting the whole of the organization be affected by their respective specific complexities. A legal department may be created to deal with legal issues; an education division to deal with the students and trainees circulating in the hospital; a finance directorate should deal with the respective payment routines, and so on. Despite critical instances where, for instance, the economic system seems to dictate what the medical teams could or could not do, the interplay of communications find the necessary solutions and functional separations; social differentiations must be maintained in accordance with the identity of the organization.

According to the theory, the differentiated sub-units in an organization can communicate with each other as they belong to the same organization. Many organizational decisions equally affect all its sub-units and are matters of concern for all of them. However, the separation of semantic areas should be maintained; accountants do not discuss and make decisions about treatments with doctors, or vice versa. However, this does not preclude a sub-unit to communicate with an equivalent sub-unit in another organization, as long as they both belong to the same *function system*. This means that finance officers, for instance, can communicate with finance officers belonging to other organizations as they are communicating within the economic system using the respective codes. The same is valid for all other function systems (education, political, scientific, religious, etc.). By this expedient architecture, organizations can overcome the limits of their operational closure and communicate with other organizations.[2]

---

[2] Comprehensive treatment of these topics can be found in T. Drepper, "Organization and Society", and D. Baecker, "The Design of Organization in Society", respectively chapters 8 and 9 of the book edited by Seidl and Becker (2006)

This chapter refers to studies from Scandinavian countries where the issue of poly-contexturality has been given attention. Key for the understanding of a poly-contextural architecture is to recognize the interplay of observations, with observers in the different domains observing each other. References for this discussion can be found in the book edited by Knudsen and Vogd (2015).

Every contexture observes its specific issues within its limited field. What is excluded from a field of observation of a contexture, if nevertheless relevant for the organization, becomes part and is observed by another one adequately equipped for carrying out the required observations. The legal department does not look into the procurement of disposable materials for the wards; nor does the nursing department get into communications about the legality of cases caught in legal quagmires. The separation of fields of observations and communication must be maintained and guaranteed inside the organization.

Yet there should not be hierarchical differences, because what each contexture executes cannot be executed by any of the others. Multiple contextures therefore coexist without distorting the fundamental autopoiesis of the organization as a healthcare organization.

For that, regulation of contextures has to be in place, ensuring that issues are addressed by the appropriate contexturality, reducing the overall internal complexity. Indeterminacy is only tolerated temporarily; decisions need to take place and the appropriate contexture identified for taking care of the issue. *Decisions premises* give predictability to these processes and stabilize expectations, reducing complexities (see Chapter 1).

There is room for the respective decisions to be taken separately by the concerned contexture. Those on the medical side who establish the diagnostics and treatments, and perform the respective operations, do not make the decisions to carry out or not specific procedures dependent on whether the patient is or isn't covered by insurance. Medical staff of the hospital communicate the treatment needs, which might require administrative authorization to go ahead. The administrative sections will ensure that the patient or the insurer will pay for the procedure (in a public sector hospital this process is often not needed). Therefore, the decision whether or not to perform the procedure is taken at different moments for different reasons by those in different positions in the organization. But the definition of the treatment the patient needs is exclusively within the realm of health communications.

When the insurer authorizes the procedure based on the doctors' recommendation, the insurer is not acting as part of the health *function system* but rather as a payer operating in the economic system, paying for the service.

Therefore, decisions concerning the use of the health/sick code (diagnosis, prescription and treatment) are taken exclusively by those operating within the frame of the health *function system* inside the health organization (hospital). Only doctors establish the treatment but the procedures may be performed after being approved by other systems (insurers from the economic system, as exemplified above).

An illustrative example of the separation of contexts is the Diagnostic-Related Group (DRG) and their pricing mechanisms. DRGs are used in relationships between healthcare providers and healthcare services payers, and are based on the separation of the two fields: On one side, medical discretion and decision-making; on the other, economic transactions involving payments. This maintains and reproduces the differentiation between the two function systems.

Poly-contexturality is widespread, reflecting the fact that systems are present in each other's environment and produce effects that are often relevant for each system individually. Hospitals have always been sites of multiple interests and multiple communications. The coupling with other function systems has, from the beginning, to be part of any endeavour to build, equip and open hospitals. Human resources have to be hired and many types of services have to be bought. Finances of some sort have to flow in to keep the organization running. Certain interactions with legal and political systems have to be constructed to allow the hospital to function in specific locations, to conform to expectations and requirements those systems may have.

So, that is not new, and existed well before commercial interests became a relevant feature of health systems. What is important to keep in mind, though, is the architecture by which poly-contexturality happens; each function system has to have its specific operations, which can only be done in their respective semantic meaningful domain, and performed within their specific organizational space.

Within the complexities of poly-contexturality, the organization's main social identity has to be and indeed is preserved. If a hospital becomes a school, a factory, a commercial enterprise, etc. losing its distinctiveness as a healthcare institution, it can no longer claim to be part of the health system. It no longer has the possibility of producing communications recognizable as legitimate deployment of the healthy/sick codes and related programmes. The health system's organizations would cease recognizing any health organization that steps over the line, and would no longer accept it as addressee for health communications.

Because of that, a hospital cannot neglect its main character, and must preserve the capacity to be observed by the health system as being part of it. That is expressed strongly in the communications of medical professionals in defence of their prerogative of being the only ones authorized to make legitimate use of the health codes and programmes (deciding and doing what a patient needs). There are strong barriers against commercial interference in medical decisions and attempts to make hospitals businesses just like any other, i.e. an enterprise for revenue and profit-making.

However, as mentioned above, it is still possible to have operational poly-contextures, as long as they do not disrupt the autopoiesis and identities that must be preserved. To manage that, the organization admits a certain differentiation of decision-making prerogatives, which are consistent with the preservation of communications and channels essential for the stability of expectations.

The coupled systems in a poly-contextural context may observe that they are dependent on each other, but at the same time also observe that their observations carry different concerns and considerations. A decision that is medically correct can be problematic from a financial or legal point of view. Similarly, a legally and financially correct decision may not be compatible with the rules of the medical profession.

Poly-contexture implicates a potential for conflicts and tensions. However the difficulties, the combination of different contextures is also needed as a solution to deal with the complexities of the environment and to prevent these complexities from overwhelming the organization itself. By being poly-contextural a hospital simultaneously reduces the complexities of its environment (selecting appropriately what it needs to deal with) and reduces its internal complexities (by selecting which internally constructed contexture will handle the pertinent issues).

A last and also advanced point of the theory on organizations and function systems differentiation deals with the fact that organizations and function systems are closely interlinked and dependent on each other. Luhmann (2007, p. 668) says; "organizations are the only social systems that can communicate with their environment", i.e. communicate with other organizations in the environment. By being able to communicate with other organizations, while preserving their individual operational closure, organizations also preserve the differentiation of the function systems, which cannot communicate with other function systems. As the codes and semantics of health are only understandable and meaningful within the context of the health function system, this system also cannot meaningfully deploy the codes belonging to other function systems. Function systems cannot organize themselves – i.e. take the form of organizations; therefore, they need organizations.

To grasp this corollary of the theory it is necessary to keep in mind that function systems are semantic universes, which only understand their specific codes; the legal system, for example, cannot communicate in the same way as communications take place inside a health system, or vice versa. Poly-contextural organization therefore reinforces social differentiation, making it possible for the organizations to perform communicative operations in different function systems. It can be said that organizations solve the problem of isolation of the function systems at the same time as preserving them, making simultaneously possible both the autopoiesis of the function systems and of the organizations as poly-contextural sites.

In short, this chapter intended to provide researchers of health organizations the conceptual tools by which they can address the complex relationships between different organizations and the internal expressions of different function systems.

Key texts (included in the references at the end of the book) in Social System Theory and organizations are: N. Thygesen (2012), *The Illusion of Management Control: A Systems Theoretical Approach to Managerial Technologies*; David Seidl and Kai Helge Becker (2006), *Niklas Luhmann and Organization Studies*; Luhmann (2018), *Organization and Decision;* Vogd and Knudsen (2015), *Systems Theory and the Sociology of Health and Illness*; M. Knudsen (2012), "Structural Coupling between Organizations and Function Systems: Looking at Standards in Health Care" (in *The Illusion of Management Control: A Systems Theoretical Approach to Managerial Technologies*, ed. by N. Thygesen); David Seidl and Hannah Mormann (2014), "Niklas Luhmann as Organization Theorist" (chapter 7 in *Oxford Handbook of Sociology, Social Theory and Organization Studies: Contemporary Currents*); Tore Bakken and Tor Hermes, eds. (2012), *Autopoietic Organization Theory*.

Chapter 8 – Critics' Views about Luhmann's Theory

This chapter gives an overview of the critics of Luhmann's theory. Like any grand theory, it is not exempt from controversy. The book lists six among the most common criticisms, giving the references and explaining the issues. However, the book does not enter into the controversies, defending or criticizing Luhmann. This chapter rather acknowledges the existing opinions and gives readers indications on how to reflect on them. Brief opinions are nevertheless expressed.

First, we give brief biographical information about Luhmann. He was born in Germany in Lüneburg in December 1927. He graduated in law and in 1960 received a scholarship to study with Talcott Parsons at Harvard University; at that time, Parsons was one of the most prominent sociologists. Luhmann was influenced by Parsons' theories and theory crafting but soon he moved on to his own formulation of sociological concepts. Some of Parsons' concepts are still found in Luhmann's work, although they often have slightly different understandings. One of these concepts is *symbolically generalized means of communication* (see the Annex). Two major influences in Luhmann's work are the mathematician George Spencer-Brown, with his work published in *The Law of Forms*, where he developed a calculus based on the drawing of distinctions for observational purposes, and the works of the biologists Varela and Maturana, who developed the concept of autopoiesis. These two sources of influence represent two major turns in the development of the Social System Theory to the final format it took from the 1980s onwards. Luhmann was remarkably productive, and during his life published around 75 books and 500 articles (Borch 2011). He worked at Bielefeld University from 1965 until his death in 1998.

Luhmann's style itself has been seen as responsible for the limited attention his theory has received; it is a writing style that often requires efforts from his readers given the complexities of the texts. However, those who manage to get through his constructions become convinced of his theory's robustness and consistency. Luhmann is considered one of the most prominent theoreticians in social science in the twentieth century. The twenty-first century has not yet revealed anyone who could claim the same prominence. Social scientists are resolute in confirming the greatness of what he has achieved and the integrity, erudition, comprehensiveness and intellectual honesty of his work.

It is important to bear in mind a few points when critically approaching the Social System Theory. Luhmann's work needs to be understood in line with its position in the philosophical perspective of what can be called constructivist realism. In that theory, both system and environment might have an ontological "nature" which nevertheless cannot be fully comprehended as to what they essentially are; the descriptions are generated by observers, who, in order to carry out observations, use the system/environment distinction.

Luhmann's constructivism therefore does not deny the existence of reality or the presence of systems and environments in that reality. However, the observation of a system, and the subsequent narratives that communicate what has been researched, will not entirely comprise or reproduce the observed objects. The narrative constructs an image of the system with the elements and relations the observations could identify and select.

There are a number of reasons for that. First, the observer would not have the *requisite variety* to represent one-to-one the points observed in the system and its environment. Neither the complexity of the environment nor of the system could be fully incorporated into the complexity of the narrative, which itself has to be formed with complexity-reducing orientation. The constructivism therefore means that the described system is a construction of the observer, but in any case, a construction that is not tautological or self-created; it has anchors in the forms of reality (causalities, where applicable) which are observed and incorporated into the narratives. The epistemological difficulties of the constructivism are further discussed and the interested reader is recommended texts where the topic has been treated at length.

We can move on to the critical points often talked about in relation to the theory:

- The theory is criticized for being too eclectic, borrowing too many concepts from different sources;
- The transposition of the term autopoiesis from its original biological science context to social science is viewed with some skepticism, including by the biologists who formulated the concept;

- Luhmann's concepts about the function of the political system are attacked from both the left and the right side of the political spectrum;
- Lack of empirical evidence – Luhmann dedicated his entire academic life to construct a theoretical edifice without having carried out empirical studies to confirm (or not) his theoretical constructs.
- The theory is criticized for not taking humans into consideration – these critics point to the fact that human beings do not appear in the theory.

We present only a brief description of the critics, except for a longer discussion on the last bullet point.

- The theory is criticized for being too eclectic, borrowing too many concepts from different sources

This does not seem to be a relevant criticism, as the borrowing itself cannot be rejected regardless of quantity. What does indeed matter is the clarity of the concepts and the coherence by which they are articulated in building the theory. Luhmann does not deal hurriedly or superficially with what he imports. Serious reflections were undertaken. Not much can be found and said if one goes about looking for loose concepts that are not meaningfully integrated into the theory.

- The transposition of the term autopoiesis from its original biological science context to social science is viewed with some skepticism, including by the biologists who formulated the concept

This controversy developed in exchanges between Maturana and Luhmann. The biologists remained sceptical in relation to the use of the concept of autopoiesis for social systems. The precision by which biological systems are separated from their environment, with concrete physical boundaries, could not replicate social systems with semantic boundaries. The transposition of autopoiesis to such a system/environment distinction requires thinking about boundaries in less concrete terms although still performing the separation function. Those who may get in touch with the term autopoiesis in the sociological context before learning it from biological texts would not have difficulties in understanding how the idea works for social systems. However the controversy exists and some readers may be interested in studying it more closely.

- Luhmann's concepts about the function of the political system are attacked from both the left and the right side of the political spectrum

This is surely a long discussion, which would require elements that have not yet been fully explained in the book. A thorough, comprehensive examination of this questions can be found in Michael King and Chris Thornhill (2003), with extensive explanations of the operations of the legal and the political systems, and comprehensive treatment of the political philosophy themes that inform the controversies.

- Lack of empirical evidence – Luhmann dedicated his entire academic life to construct a theoretical edifice without having carried out empirical studies to confirm (or not) his theoretical constructs

Luhmann did not carry out empirical assessment and data collection to demonstrate the concepts and the relations between them. Luhmann's work was essentially theoretical and concerned with the validity and soundness of the conceptual construction. This does not mean that the concepts were detached from reality and existed in an imaginary world; of course not. The conceptualization, while still dealing with abstractions and generalization, was grounded in solid reflections on the real empirical possibility of their existence. Any statement that the theory is not concerned with social reality is a hasty conclusion, at its best showing a lack of understanding of the theory.

- The theory is criticized for not taking humans into consideration – these critics point to the fact that human beings do not appear in the theory

For this point, we need to try to provide a longer explanation. We briefly discuss the theoretical constructs some readers might find difficult to grasp. When explaining the work of the systems, Luhmann often uses metaphors implying the existence of a "self" communicating and making the decisions at the core of the system. That can be a difficult point, which can be associated with criticism of the "lack" of humans in the processes of the systems. However, such an impression is superficial. A careful consideration of the role of communication and the capacity of communication to interlace with other communications, constructing scenarios and narratives that may not entirely represent what any of the participants in the communication specifically have in mind, is key to understanding the question. Communication can be viewed as having a life "independent" from those engaged in it. It is important to grasp how that can be the case.

Communication is essential in the constitution of the social. It is what makes the social possible. However, communication is not equal to what is in the mind of those who communicate; in Luhmann's thinking, communication does not carry any fundamental validity for communicating essentially truthful rational statements or the complete picture one has in mind. Partial comprehension and misunderstanding are as likely to be the result of communication as of understanding.

Luhmann's project clashed with Habermas' views in a debate that unfolded over two decades of exchanges between the two (see Borch 2011, p. 120, and King and Thornhill 2003, p. 165). Having himself developed a theory of the social based on communication, Habermas (2007) criticized Luhmann's position, exposing the differences between the theoretical perspectives. This book does not cover the full discussion, however some points will be helpful for readers to reach their own conclusions in relation to the assumed "self" that is at the core of the "self-referenced" and "self-organizing" systems of Social Systems Theory.

Habermas represents a modern school of thought for which the possibility of intersubjectivity shaping overarching common rationalities is a better explanation of the social than the independence of functional systems, constructing their own individual rationalities. Habermas' project firmly believes in the achievement of final truthful agreement between the parts once the "ideal speech situation" for social communications is exercised.

The belief in the possibility of internal connection, inscribed in the ontological inner nature of rational meanings and communications, is in clear contrast with social systems understanding of the possibilities of communication, as putting forward contingent selections the systems are interested and able to make at the communications junctures.

In contrast with the Habermasian approach, validity is attributable to what looks valid and can be agreed upon as such by those capable and motivated to communicate about it. The obvious validity of the non-existence of an elephant in the room does not require even two fully self-conscious adults discussing the matter; a couple of four-year-old kids would reach such a conclusion on the validity of the judgement with expressive communication between them. On the other hand, on matters of values, interpretations of facts or motivations a lot more is required. But still, validity is not part of the essence of the statements; it is only part of the assumptions and wished for expectations that can be agreed upon. Meanings are contingent and can be different, no matter the truthfulness and faithfulness of those communicating.

Arising out of a confusion about what Social System Theory actually says, some readers may struggle to accept the role of communication as the system's building block, assuming that this would imply accepting the idea of communication "simulating" or "concocting" a kind of "virtual self", with similar decision-making and self-reflection attributes, as the "selves" of conscious individuals engaged in communication. As mentioned above, Luhmann's metaphors may induce such confusion; however, we admit, the metaphors help the intuition of the system's self-reference and self-reproduction.

Self-reproduction is but the system, "anchored" on the memories of those communicating, bringing back, processing, adjusting and upholding concepts and semantics previously selected as constitutive of the system. The memories of the psychic systems (the minds) actualize the elements that can then be confirmed, maintained, changed or discarded as representing legitimate communications of the system. Luhmann's metaphors imply these understandings.

For example, when Luhmann (2013, p. 64) says: "a system does not operate [communicate] in the environment", this does not mean that the "self" of the system makes the decision not to communicate. This statement becomes clear if we consider that communication involves the two parts making utterances with their respective contents, leading to recursive understanding (or misunderstanding). The environment does not make utterances. If those communicating are understandably deploying the codes of the system, they are communicating inside the system; or, better still, their communication is part of the system in contrast with the environment.

If there are utterances perceived as coming from the environment, those are due to the presence of another system (psychic or social) in the environment, producing them. If the utterances carry relevant recognizable meanings for the observing system (as when a doctor asks a patient about what he feels and the patient communicates the location of the discomfort), they are observed and processed, becoming information inside the system, and then incorporated in the respective semantic fields of meanings the system recognizes as of interest.

Furthermore, communication can always: 1) follows the path intended by one of the participants; or 2) the path intended by more than one of those engaged; or 3) neither of the paths described in 1 and 2, thus generating results that might be unsatisfactory for all involved. In such case, the communication seems to follow its own path, determined by associations or links of ideas and semantics that are not in anyone's plans, with deviances that are not detected or successfully corrected by those involved.

Communicatively, undesirable results thus reached arise out of communications' own predicaments, but still cannot be said to reveal a "self"-driven intention by some sort of "selfless self". Surely none of the engaged consciences were able to successfully strategize the argumentation in those unsuccessful communications.

A metaphor can straightforwardly convey the idea of the system's self-observation and self-reference and its final decision of self-organization, as if a transcendent self was fully conscious of the processes and in charge of the decision-making. As if such a self could act independently from the conscious selves of the individuals communicating. This is obviously the metaphor's effect; there is no such meta-conscience in the Social System Theory, or transcendental self, or unconscious invariant structures at work, as would be the preference of the structuralisms of the last century. The self-reference metaphor conveys well the idea that communication follows paths that are not entirely under the control of either of the parts involved, and in that, metaphoricaly, "it has a life of its own".

On the other hand, it is important to keep in mind that there would be no systems' communications and decisions if there were no psychic systems (selves) communicating and communicatively reaching decisions. The communications could not exist independently from psychic systems as, in other words, there would not be any social systems without the individuals communicating inside them. Putting this differently, a system cannot do without the individuals communicating in it. Any attempt to discredit Social Systems Theory for radically separating the systems and the individuals, and seeing them as having entirely independent lives, is a misrepresentation of the theory.

To be clear, communication opens a range of possible outcomes. Within the field of possibilities, selections made over the course of the communications (selections that are communicated and then accepted or not, affecting subsequent communications) construct the path the communication "walks". Implicitly or explicitly, selections are communicated and communicatively accepted or rejected. Although still unpredictable from the start, the conclusion will remain within the range of the possible, if one could carry out the difficult task to map out all possibilities of sequences from the start.

Because a comprehensive mapping would be too complex to be reasonably established, the unfolding of the communication may develop in unpredictable ways. One may say that "evil" or "angelic" inspirations brought the communication to its final conclusion, as if a self was overseeing the whole process from above. Such explanations are obviously only poetical metaphors to express judgements about the final outcome of the communications.

A grasp of the operations of this metaphoric "selfless self" of communications is a pivotal point to understand systems from the Social Systems Theory perspective. Despite Habermas' discomfort,[1] one does not need to struggle to accept this notion and its usefulness for better understanding of social systems based on communications. Even with its contingent selections and non-essential validity of communicated statements, communication can indeed be the only phenomenon to explain the build-up of social systems.

A final point, also arriving from the polemic between Luhmann and Habermas, the theme of intersubjectivity deserves some reflections. Although Luhmann used the term "interpenetration" in his early theoretical constructions, he later opted for the notion of "structural coupling" to explain stable relationships between two operationally closed but interconnected systems, whereby they nevertheless preserve their operational closure.[2]

Communication does not require intersubjectivity; ego and alter, two psychic systems, using the same language and the same sets of signs and meanings, reach common understanding of statements, which they may communicatively confirm. Ego may ask whether alter agrees with his understanding of the statements alter had just uttered. By confirming their agreement, both can rely on that mutual understanding and move on to subsequent statements.

No intersubjective event is required to explain this agreement process; the minds remain isolated in their own self-references, and the differentiation between the two is not trespassed. It can be easily accepted that the complexities that each mind manages (with all the selections it processes) would be too

---

1   One may say, on Habermas, that validity claims are rarely fully rationally activated in the processes of communication.
2   In *Social Systems* Luhmann (1995) dedicated chapter 6 to the interpenetration topic. He explains that the notion should not be equated to the input–output relation model, but rather, in his words, "we speak of 'penetration' if a system makes its own complexities (and with it indeterminacy, contingency and the pressure to select) available for constructing another system" (Luhmann 1995, p. 213), while remaining an environment for each other. This happens reciprocally, he adds, as for instance in relationships between psychic and social systems, where the complexities of the psychic system involved in the deployment of utterance and information actively construct the complexities of the communications of the social system.

heavy a burden for any other mind to incorporate into its own complexity, considering that it would be keeping up with the selection it makes itself.

Intersubjectivity is thus a useless concept, although the aspiration of its occurrence can still be hoped for. One can have strong beliefs about someone else's intentions and feelings, but those will remain "hypothetical", even in the face of an explicit admission by the other of his true intents. Language usage cannot be fenced against the possibility of convincingly lying.

The key references consulted for critical analysis of Luhmann's work are: M. King and C. Thornhill (2003); Hans-Georg Moeller (2005, 2012); C. Borch (2011); W. Rasch (2000); D. Seidl and H. Mormann (2014); Habermas (2007); and L. Leydesdorff (2002). Details are provided in the references section of the book.

Chapter 9 – Prospects and Examples

Having presented the theory in the previous chapters, its application to health systems, and methodological issues, this chapter gives examples of the use of the theory to assess interventions, research and development projects. The examples were taken from publications in the health systems literature and projects in which the author was involved.

With international development aid's continuous attention to health systems thinking and health systems strengthening, it is necessary to review the paradigms by which health systems have so far been approached. Concepts such as autopoiesis and operational closure acknowledge social systems' autonomy and vital dynamics for their existence and reproduction. Researchers, observing health systems (from inside or outside) need to realize that systems are not amenable to interventions that do not recognize their autonomous and self-organizing nature. They are often confronted with realities that lead them to acknowledge that the systems are active in the selection of what is relevant for them. Observers, who are not part of the system, and therefore do not participate in the autopoiesis of the system and its organizations, cannot solve the problems. Even if aid is needed, provided and welcome, only the system can put it to good use. Detached from ideological orientations, the theory gives substantive arguments in this direction.

From the literature, 12 texts were selected and are presented as examples of how Social Systems Theory can offer new insights on the respective health system topics. The articles and reports were chosen for the relevance of the themes in the current international health context. Several constructs of the Social Systems Theory are used, particularly the central concepts: autopoiesis, self-reference, observation, communication, differentiation, operational closure, complexity, organization, decision-making, etc. Given the scope of this book, the texts present summary discussions. Particular attention is given to three of the texts, which are discussed in more detail.

9.1 Dual practices

Health professionals' double employment links (usually one job in the public sector and another in the private sector) and remuneration are the topics of a paper by L. Paina et al. (2014) focusing on Uganda. The paper concludes that, despite government efforts to prevent or control dual practices, they linger on because public and private sector incentives, financial and non-financial alike, are complementary and health professionals find ways of carrying on with them. Agreeing with the presented empirical evidences, Social System Theory analysis would take into account the relevance of membership and the decision-making prerogatives for autopoiesis of the organizations with which the health professionals establish their dual links. In both public and private entities the professional members are participants in the autopoietic reproduction of the organizations. They maintain that the duality does not compromise the autopoiesis of the individual organization of which they are members. In that sense, dual practices are issues that the *function system* and healthcare provider organizations do not need to care much about. Dual practices are not self-referentially problematized into the service provider *organizations* carrying out their individual reproduction. As long as the professionals come along and perform a "fair deal" regarding the expected duties, there is no need to pressure them to follow more strictly their contracts and associated expectations. The health organizations know well that health professionals are scarce and not readily available in the labour market. The political system (a distinct function system compared to the health system) instead, responding to the media and to pressures external to the health system, tries to intervene. This is described in Paina et al.'s paper. However, the political system does not succeed in influencing the reproductive dynamics of the health organizations. Public and private healthcare service provider organizations are not, jointly or individually, under the same pressure to address the issue as the political system is. However, as is usually the case in political systems, topics have a short life span and are soon replaced by emergent issues that capture public attention and shift the pressures on the politicians to focus on the new topics. Often the political system enacts policies or legal instruments and moves on to other concerns without assuring proper follow-up and implementation of past decisions. This is also well described in the paper, which narrates empirical observations on how managers adapt to the dual practices. The theory would foresee such an outcome by considering the way the health and political systems as well as public and private organizations work as autopoietic operationally closed systems.

9.2 Accreditation of health facilities

Attempts to introduce accreditation of health facilities is likely to face difficulties and perhaps insurmountable barriers if they do not pay attention to the self-observation and self-organization capabilities of organizations, and the vital importance of these functions in their self-reference. In this regard, accreditation is a suitable topic for an analysis of self-observation. Accreditation sets standards to be adopted as references for internal and/or external evaluation of healthcare service providers. It requires and implies that the provider refers and communicates about itself using the language and terms the accreditation evaluation guidelines prescribe. Without a self-reference perspective, accreditation initiatives and studies do not apprehend the core dynamic of the process. An example of that is the article on accreditation practices in Kerala, India, by Sindhu Joseph (2021). It reports on a cross-sectional study including accredited (312) and non-accredited (309) primary (community health centre) and secondary (general, women and children, and small hospitals) public healthcare facilities. According to the article, a questionnaire asked patients' views on ten dimensions: physical facility, admission services, patient centredness, accessibility of medical care, financial matters, professionalism, staff services, medical quality, diagnostic services and patient satisfaction. The answers were given on a 5-point scale (1 = strongly agree to 5 = strongly disagree). The results showed that the median score of dimensions of accredited primary healthcare facilities in the structure, process and outcome domains are higher than for the non-accredited hospitals. The study also found significant differences between the scores for these same three domains in accredited and non-accredited primary healthcare institutions but absent in secondary care institutions. The paper concludes that the accreditation process needs to be improved. Social System Theory would call our attention to the observers. The researchers as observers of observers could choose between inquiring into the patients or the professionals – two different sets of observers with surely different perspectives. The researchers, external observers themselves, would need to realize that the communications established with patients and/or staff have different structures. Staff possibly would not be interested in revealing sensitive information related to accreditation processes to an external observer; and patients would have biased, perhaps poorly informed, understanding of the issues at stake in the assessed dimensions. Social System Theory provides valuable orientation for such assessments.

9.3 Check-up programme in Albania

This example is a reflection on how political decisions taken by the political system may not be in line with health systems strengthening, as the Systems Theory would see it. The Ministry of Health implemented a compulsory medical check-up programme for a segment of the adult population in Albania. The programme defined the exams in the routine check-up without doctors making decisions on the individual laboratory and other exams to request. By introducing a pre-defined set of exam prescriptions, the programme removed the prerogatives of the medical doctors to decide on what the patient actually needed (or not) based on clinical evaluations of the patients. Not all patients would be required to undergo the same examinations, if that decision depended exclusively on the doctors' observation of indicative signs of possible disorders and needs of further investigation. The resources wasted on unnecessary examinations could have been used instead for appropriate follow-up of symptomatic patients or those who had already started treatment. In that regard, with the excuse of offering a comprehensive check-up for all citizens over 45 years of age, the programme in fact took away from the medical professionals some of their otherwise standard procedure of ordering examinations. The reduction in the prerogatives of the health professionals to make all decisions concerning every individual patient represents a decrease in the level of complexity that the health system was already perfectly capable of taking responsibility for. This demonstrates how the de-differentiation of the two distinct functional systems, the political and the health systems, can have negative effects on the system that in consequence loses the scope of its distinct prerogatives. The conclusion to be drawn here is that the Ministry of Health, a participant in the political system to a greater extent than it is a participant in the health system, has the themes of the communications of the political system closer to its core concerns than the actual communications delivering the health codes in diagnostic and treatment contexts. The example is based on direct experience of the author while managing a project to strengthen the primary healthcare service provision in the country, and was published in a local newspaper.

9.4 Universal Health Cover (UHC)

This example uses Social System Theory to reflect on political system approaches to health systems concerns in a globalized context; the discussion does not focus on any specific paper however. The intention is to bring to the fore the differences in the perspectives of political players communicating at international level and those communicating in the actual operations of the health systems at country level. The argument is that the need to set new semantics and orientation of communications in the international arena differs from the needs of decision-makers dealing with the limits in the capacity of their countries' public health systems to tackle actual health problems in the context of the structures they already have in place. We refer to the differentiation of two distinct functional systems (political and health), where the problems concerning the political international players are not the same as the health systems on the ground have to cope with. An impressionist portrayal of this configuration would picture two independent "parallel universes" of communications, pursuing their unconnected individual reproduction, while trying to have some influence on each other. While in the political system the political legitimacy and general acceptance of the themes and decisions are at stake, in the country's health system, the daily reproduction of the medical communications and related actions has the unquestionable priority. The complexities addressed by these two systems are also very different. Policy-making at international level requires complex communications among various interests – complexity reduction in this context aims at narrowing down the sets of meaningful themes that can be commonly addressed and reasonably understood and shared. The complexity reduction for the health system "on the ground" consists in reproducing the communications that are already redundant (i.e. with established, stable meanings) while guardedly incorporating new meanings. Successes in these two "parallel universes" are measured differently; while in international politics, governments signing official declarations, incorporating some of the UHC semantics in policy documents and official speeches, is already counted as success, even if these changes in communications at the level of political systems do not translate into corresponding changes at health systems level. By fully adopting UHC promises to provide all healthcare needed by anyone, a public health system brings the full weight of complexities to its table. This presents an overwhelming challenge, and health systems are uninterested in getting too bogged down in operational and pragmatic terms, or effectively try to comprehensively deliver. Although a valid horizon to be reached in an undetermined future, the achievements can be only and perhaps frustratingly partial. The main argument presented in this section is that while UHC works well at the level of international macro-political agreements, it is destined to fail at implementation level because of unreachable targets. Here Social Systems Theory would emphasize the need to pay attention to the domains of communications and the observers operating in them.

9.5 Governance and informal payments

This example discusses a case of autopoiesis orienting the way a health system finds solutions for its survival. The example focuses on Tajikistan, where a public health system surviving a civil war in the midst of government collapse, informally adopted practices to carry on working independently from government funds. The health system survived with the incorporation of informal payments into its normal functioning. The health facilities were not maintained; the government could not do that. Salaries were sometimes not paid for months. To retain minimal working conditions, health staff had to contribute part of the money collected from patients. These practices remained in place well after the end of the civil war, while the government budget continued to be too low to pay salaries, maintain structures and equipment, and make badly needed investment. Health professionals regularly communicated among themselves about the solutions they adopted, and it was not uncommon for part of the health facilities' and wards' informal revenues to be passed up through the hierarchy to higher ranks, who left these informal practices undisturbed, despite the laws against it. The governance thus in place reflected the prevailing systemic autopoietic drive, in spite of non-conformity with formal legal rules in place, and the protests of the international donors supporting the government. This example is based on three years of direct experience of the author while living in the country and managing a donor-funded project to strengthen primary healthcare, along with publications in the literature on informal payment in Central Asia.

9.6 Health systems strengthening

This section reflects on the possibilities to strengthen a self-referential system with the characteristics of operational closure, self-organization, autopoiesis, and constructed by communications. In addition to the extensive theoretical discussions in Chapter 6, this example focuses on the article by J. Goldberg and M. Bryant (2012). This article was picked up among many others for the opportunity to discuss two important notions in heath development aid, country ownership and capacity building. As stated by the title of the article, "Country Ownership and Capacity Building: The Next Buzzwords in Health Systems Strengthening or a Truly New Approach to Development?", it tries to figure out how these strategic orientations can deliver strengthened health systems. The terms "country ownership" had come to prominence after high-profile meetings of aid donors sponsoring health systems development in developing countries. The Paris Declaration on Aid Effectiveness (2005) was a watershed, after which country ownership firmly entered the development aid discourse of most donors and international agencies. "Country ownership' implied a change in donors' postures and actions, and predominantly the determination to use country mechanisms for implementing aid projects, using their finance structures, their political decision-making as well as public sector managerial institutions. In this sense, the term comes close to acknowledgement of the concept of autopoiesis, understood as systems' production of the means for their own reproduction. However, the two notions are not equivalent and differ in many respects. The crucial difference is that there is no alternative to autopoiesis, which implies that only the system can take care of itself, while "country ownership" still suggests that something can be or was different before the agenda was established, or, in other words, the health systems of the developing country did not own all its programmes. As matter of fact, aid was (and may still is) often channelled directly to some types of provision of care without the involvement or even awareness of the governments. By the time of the Paris declaration, it became clear that such uncoordinated ways of supporting developing countries were wasteful and ineffective. For example, Ministries of Health were losing qualified staff and competences for donor projects, becoming therefore less able to run their own organizations. Regardless of these acute shortcomings, though, the autopoiesis of public health organizations and of health as a function system did not stop. We will come back to this point. "Capacity building" is the provision of training and working conditions for the health workforce in managerial, service delivery or any other position. Although initially carried out independently, "capacity building", as advocated by the authors of the article, should enhance competences to increase the possibility of "country ownership"; this is how the two terms connect. Without improved competences, it is implied, "country ownership" will not happen. On the other hand, "capacity building" is a field of initiatives where "country ownership" can be exercised and made operational; "country owned capacity building" should be the new paradigm, the authors propose.

Using the Social Systems Theory concept of complexity, "country ownership" and "capacity building" orient donors' supports towards making public systems of aid-recipient countries able to deal with the complexities of running larger and more diverse initiatives; the countries would be expected to reach the stage where they could run new initiatives by their own means. In line with the notion of autopoiesis of the Social Systems Theory, this enhancement of capacity to deal with increased complexities fairly translates the notion of systems strengthening. However, autopoiesis implies that the system is the only one that can decide about itself. This theoretical perspective pushes further the notion of country ownership, beyond what development aid assumes. Autopoiesis means that the existing systems have always been the owners of what they do. Before the Paris declaration donors carried out their business as they wanted, and the public system tolerated, accepted and incorporated lack of coordination into their own strategies, even if not explicitly stated. Eventually donors realized they were not achieving much by doing the work themselves, and also understood that real development would require operations to be performed by the governments themselves. That indeed increased the awareness about government capabilities. However, as consideration of autopoiesis highlights, an autopoietic system would only advance by its own self-reproductive capabilities. Funds can come from abroad, but the communications the systems sustain can only be reproduced by the systems' mechanisms. Governments were only interested in taking responsibility up to the point they saw the advantages and considered they had the ability to do so. They would not overtax themselves with tasks beyond their capacities and above the level of effort they could deploy. By being able to conduct self-observation, self-referential systems (including here health and political systems and their organizations) have identities regarding what they are and what they can and want to do (or not) – this is how self-organization is possible. In short, autopoiesis and self-reference were and are constantly at work, although donors were not paying attention and often felt frustrated with lack of success or willingness of the governments to follow what donors thought they could and should have done. Lack of understanding of autopoiesis was and still is a problem for the whole development aid enterprise. Some progress has been achieved though, as donors started to adopt the principle of "government in the driving seat", and developed trust and reliance on aid modalities such as budget support, by which money was transferred to the country's treasury without being earmarked for specific projects, and the government would only subscribe to jointly agreed sets of indicators, targets and reporting mechanisms; everything else, including operational decisions and implementation, was in the government's hands. This is indeed more in line with what Social System Theory would recommend. But one should not lose focus on the operational closures, by which both government institutions and donors' organizations communicate internally about observations that each independently performs using the semantics that are relevant for each one's self-references. This may still create gaps in communication between the organizations that are difficult to bridge.

9.7 Mother and child health (MCH)

The author was involved with the implementation of a donor's support to a MCH programme in Guinea Bissau, where a package of benefits for health workers and pregnant women was introduced (the work was communicated in several internal consultancy reports). The package intended to terminate the user fees charged to pregnant women during antenatal care and at delivery. It was expected that health workers would be compensated for the payments they would no longer receive from the patients, and the pregnant women would be motivated to demand care as consultations, medicines and maternity care would be free of charge. The expected outcome was a reduction in maternal and infant mortality, of which Guinea-Bissau had one of the highest rates in the world. In social systems terms, the changes would imply the introduction of a new range of communication styles and semantics. The communications between health workers and patients and health workers among themselves would have to reflect the new set-up, where charging patients would not be acceptable. Such change in communication patterns and continuous provision of information to professionals and beneficiaries on the new arrangements would have to be achieved and maintained. In short, the programme introducing the new benefit package had also to be accompanied by information and communication strategies to ensure the new meanings circulated and were understood by all concerned. Nevertheless, there was not much attention to the communications, and the dissemination of information about the new benefits was not systematically conducted and/or evaluated. Even where and when efforts in that regard were spent, professionals and patients were used to status quo that had existed for decades, and scepticism over the continuity and sustainability of the new initiative was prevalent. We would say that patterns of communication, as well as the conditions they correspond to, are resilient (negative resilience perhaps), and the organizations and entities involved in changing them need to strategically approach the communication theme.

9.8 The fallacy of embedding research

The chapter by J. Olivier et al. (2017) advocates that health systems research should be embedded in the systems studied. This is presented as an approach, not a research method. Without getting into discussion of the previous contributions on matters of imbeddedness in the fields of sociological and anthropological methods from decades ago, our concern here is directed towards the understanding of systems that the approach overlooks. The authors optimistically say that the nearness of researchers and the system they study has advantages of more direct access to key components of the system; moreover, that makes the implementation of the study's conclusions more likely. On the other hand, the authors warn about hiccups, as the same closeness may have the disadvantage of restricting the researchers' critical views and freedom for making recommendations. In the discussion of this study our arguments highlight first that the recommended approach is a generic quasi-normative guideline for many studies in social science and public health, and it does not carry with it any specific view of what a system, or a health system, for that matter, is. We highlight the importance of having a better understanding of how systems are capable of self-reference and self-organization. Systems can carry out self-observations and make decisions for self-reproduction while preserving operational closure. Organizations, as a type of system, distinguish between members and non-members on the basis of their entitlement, respectively, to participate in decisions or not. In line with operational closure, external researchers, i.e. non-members of the organization they study, are therefore not incorporated into decision-making communications. Provision of advice, which can later be (or not) the object of consideration in decision-making circles, is the most an external observer can do. The closure is of vital importance for the survival of any organization. Yet an internal researcher, if speaking from a member's position, can be dealt with as such by the organization, which will recognize the position from which the researcher communicates. But the researcher will have to adjust communications to the semantics and channels used by the organization and their position in it. Still, being an internal researcher does not per se guarantee acceptance of the findings, even when communicated in the semantics the organization recognizes and accepts. In addition, embedding research needs to be considered in reference to social systems differentiation – for instance, health and science. An individual whose main engagement is with organizations of one of these systems is not recognized by organizations of the other system as a member with the same entitlement to communications. A scientist will communicate in terms that, although fully understandable in the context of the science system, are not entirely understood or considered relevant for those who do not belong to that system. In conclusion, the insertion of any communication in the decision-making of an organization (as a system) has to happen according to the terms and criteria the organization sets. The unawareness of this aspect leads to the creation of false expectations. Embedding therefore cannot be a guarantor of unbiased unrestricted access to information and acceptance of research conclusions by the studied system. Although it can be recommended from an ethical (quasi-normative) perspective, it still cannot assure good understanding of a system's operations and accomplishments. As a matter of cautious, modest awareness, it is better to acknowledge that the system knows and can better understand what and why it does what it does than the external researchers trying to understand it.

9.9 Voucher schemes in Tanzania and Ghana

The discussions about the article mentioned below in this example are drawn in reference to the concepts of systems' internal and external differentiation according to the Social System Theory. The article presents historical narratives of the implementation of insecticide-treated bed nets (ITN) programmes as part of the strategies for fighting malaria in Tanzania and Ghana (de Savigny et al. 2012):

> In Tanzania, vouchers have moved beyond the planning agenda, had policies and programmes formulated, been sustained in implementation at national scale for many years and have become as of 2012 the main and only publicly supported continuous delivery system for ITNs. In Ghana national-scale implementation of vouchers never progressed beyond consideration on the agenda and piloting towards formulation of policy; and the approach was replaced by mass distribution campaigns with less dependency on or integration with the health system. By 2011, Ghana entered a phase with no publicly supported continuous delivery system for ITNs. (p. 1)

If analysed from the social system perspective, the voucher schemes were not entirely part of the health systems. They were to a large extent part of the economic system, with communications and closely related economic transactions, and with the public health sub-system having some oversight and concerns related to disease risk prevention. Communications regarding the voucher schemes are not based on the health/sick code. Their associated communications represent communication with the code distinction paying/not paying for the voucher and adjusted discounted price. Once classified as pregnant and therefore entitled to the voucher, a woman would leave the health system and enter the economic system, even with the vouchers being provided inside the health facility. So, analysis of the progress of the scheme have to treat it as belonging to the economic system and related to the autopoiesis of the economic organizations involved, not the health organizations. The history of the start and subsequent development stages of the two schemes is a narrative of how the public sector came together with private partners and donors in a coupling initiative. Their economic interests and visions in the two schemes were different, which may help to understand to some extent the relatively different successes. The article would sit well as a study of public sector management and the context and results of strategic decisions. Still, it would not be dealing with health systems prerogatives of communications. Therefore, this article can be thought of as being alongside the political system and/or the economic system, with some couplings (as mothers were given vouchers in health centres) with the health system. To present a public health system perspective, it would be necessary to address issues of health risks and include health outcomes indicators, assessing the success or failure of the schemes in epidemiological terms. According to Social Systems Theory, the economic system is made up of communications that are coded as payments/nonpayments. Once a payment is made, as controversial as this may sound, the consequences that follow from the acquisition of the goods or services would no longer belong to the economic system. Communications on whether the bed nets were taken home and placed as recommended, and whether people slept under them, and so on, to ensure the preventive effectiveness of the net, would be matters for communication within the public health sub-system, assessing disease risks and the results of health programmes.

9.10 Community health workers (CHW)

The discussion in this section focuses on a paper by K. Scott, A. George and R. Ved (2019) that reports on a review of 122 articles published in India about CHW programmes. The paper sets up a framework for assessing CHW from several perspectives, including the connections between CHW programmes and the health system. The paper classified the reviewed articles according to the CHW topic they focused on and according to the relevant contents for assessments of CHW in the public health system context, in line with the proposed framework. Therefore, the paper has a wealth of insights on the operations of CHW programmes, and also reveals notions of the health system in the background, informing the review. The purpose of this section is to show that the assessment of CHW would be stronger if it was informed by an understanding of how CHW operate from the Social Systems Theory point of view, considering how CHW are placed in the central communications, self-reference and self-organizing functions of health systems.

From a Social Systems Theory perspective, CHW are viewed according to the following 15 points:

1. CHW programmes are part of the public health sub-system of a health system.
2. These programmes therefore should be seen as observed by that system as part of itself (self-observation), contributing therefore to the autopoiesis of both the health system as a whole and public health as a sub-system.
3. Communications among the CHWs and between CHWs and other members of the public health sub-system and health service provision sub-system happen inside the health system, and are valued, controlled, directed, observed, etc. as inherent to the reproduction of the public health sub-system.

4. The communities the CHWs serve are part of the environment of the public health sub-system; they are not members of the system, but are outside it.
5. In consequence of 4, the public health sub-system may need to enter into some sort of coupling with the communities to create and sustain conditions for programme implementation. Communities that set up some level of organization are potentially in a better position to enter into coupling. This leads to the drawing of a distinction between organized communities and communities of people living in the same space but without any organizational links between them.
6. For each of those roughly speaking two types of communities, the coupling will have to be different. We focus now on the organized ones.
7. An organized community does have internal observers and does observe itself pursuing its own autopoiesis. It uses the mechanisms of decisions as the basis of its communications. It makes decisions concerning its expectations about the CHW and the public health sub-system. Decisions lead to subsequent decisions and so on, reproducing the organization's expectations and observations of CHW and related communications.
8. The decisions, effective or not, followed or not, are in any case relevant for the continued decisions to be made about the presence, work, capabilities of and collaboration with the CHW.
9. These decisions are prerogatives of the organized community and are seen by itself as key to the autopoiesis of the organization they maintain.
10. The coupling of the community with the public health subsystem has also considerations related to the political system and its approaches to the community. The community, for example, may use opportunities brought about by elections to advance its objectives.
11. The observers in the public health subsystem and the observers in the communities see the CHW differently; they understand differently the relevance and capabilities of the CHW. They develop different expectations, and these expectations may be fulfilled or disappointed for different reasons, judged according to different standards of values and performance judgement criteria.
12. The narrative created by the public health sub-system to describe a successful (or failed) programme might differ largely from the narrative the community may create about the success or failure of the same programme. Furthermore, academic narratives with scientific observations and analysis of the programmes also differ from both the community's and public health sub-system's narratives.

13. The construction of the narratives uses the respective codes relevant for the respective systems, organizations and sub-systems involved. The public health sub-system uses the health-risk/non-health-risk codes with epidemiological and service provision indicators. This sub-system ultimately wants to know whether perceived health risks have been addressed by the programmes and somehow reduced. The observations have to be communicated inside the sub-system itself and then outside it to the concerned healthcare service provision sub-system (where appropriate), and, furthermore, to the political system when possible and necessary.
14. The community itself is not a system; it does not have a specific code to elaborate its communications. However, where the community establishes a representative organization, the organization communicates inside itself in accordance with membership and decision-making. Decisions are taken with the drawn distinctions used for making the respective observations. The organized community selects its distinctions based on its repertoire of distinctions it regularly uses. In that way, the organized community is able to say whether the CHWs have fulfilled completely, partially or none of the expectations.
15. The public health sub-system and the organized community may disagree radically on the way they assess the results of the CHW's activities. But they may also use references that have similar meanings for both.

By conducting an assessment of CHW programmes along these lines, a more precise perspective of community/CHW relations and possible outcomes as well as their relation with the public health sub-system can be achieved. This orientation can be summarized in the following list of guiding questions:

A) Where and who are the observers (Inside communities? Among CHW? In the public health subsystem? In the healthcare service provision subsystem? In the academic/scientific system?).
B) Are we dealing with autopoietic systems, sub-systems or organizations?
C) If yes, what is the basis of their autopoiesis?
D) Is the assessment of the programmes part of the self-observation of the sub-system and organization involved?
E) Are the communications of self-observations being incorporated into decision-making and/or interlacing with subsequent communication operations in the sub-systems and organizations involved?
F) Are CHW communications themselves being observed and assessed?

G) Is there more than one system involved in the observations (organization, sub-system or system)?
H) Have the sub-systems and organizations involved entered into structural coupling?
I) What are the codes of communication employed internally by each sub-system and/or organization involved?
J) Does the structural coupling involve communications between sub-systems and organizations?
K) On what basis do the coupled sub-systems and organizations communicate with each other? Are the codes common and share similar meanings? Or are they different?

For the content review of the 122 selected publications, the article proposed a framework with several areas of CHW programs observation: inputs, outcomes, impact, governance, interface with communities, social profile of CHW and health service context. In relation to health systems, the article classified the publications according to:

> We considered an article to have taken a health systems perspective if it examined health systems elements, such as supervision, training, supply chain management, financing, motivation, etc., or if the article discussed linkages or repercussions between health systems dimensions such as how communities supported ASHAs or whether facility providers were responsive to ASHAs. (p. 3)[1]

This shows the difficulty in approaching health systems without a firm reference of what a system is. The approaches resort to managerial (supply chain management, financing), operational (supervision), organizational (training, motivation), structural (facility providers responsibility) and functional (community support) aspects that do not necessarily and specifically reflect systemic features. For such endeavour, we propose that the key systems' aspects that need to be observed are: self-observation, self-reference, self-organization, operational closure, system/environment distinction, etc. as presented in previous chapters.

The authors of the paper looked for a number of aspects of CHW/health systems interface in the reviewed articles, which they say were rarely discussed. These were:

---

1 Accredited Social Health Activist (ASHA).

In particular, there was little consideration of programme governance (programme oversight and guidance, CHW political support, the role of NGO actors in CHW policy, grievance redressal for CHWs, programme financing and CHW programme reporting, community voice, community engagement in ASHA selection, and community collaboration with ASHAs through health committees (p. 12).

In addition, they say that more research is required to truly understand the programme as an "integrated member of the health system". These observations suggest the reviewers had expectations about the programme's autonomy and self-reliance set at a higher level than seen in a public health sub-system programme among many others

There were also expectations that the programmes would fulfil roles and achieve results wider in scope and beyond what the programme could deliver. It seems that, in the review, expectations configured objectives that were superimposed on the actual responsibilities and directionality of the CHW as a public health programme. For example: "research on other aspects of the CHW–health system framework will be increasingly important to the programme's capacity to adapt, sustain and achieve its broader goals around *empowerment, community engagement and change across the social determinants of health*" (p. 12).

These purposes can be the subject of controversies, and interpreted as political and/or ideological discourses motivated by the intention to capture or use the programmes according to the wishes of specific agendas, independently from the services delivered on the ground by those programmes. Additionally, "on-going research is required ... on realizing the *ASHA role as a community change agent, and on the influence of health system decentralization, social accountability and governance.*" (p. 12)

From a critical view informed by the Social System Theory, the survival and maintenance of the programme based on the communications it can sustain in its daily operations is a matter of the public health sub-system's reproduction, in other words, its reason for existence. "Community change', "empowerment", "decentralization" and "social accountability" are examples of the semantics of political intentions detached from the operational (health service delivery field support, disease prevention and outreach) aspects and justifications of the programme as a public health programme. The identity of the public health sub-system is at stake in the programmes it defines and implements.

It might be appropriate to point out that the position of the observer needs to be considered. An observer from the academic world has concerns and communicates in channels of the science system where that observer is inserted. The academic articles communicate differently from the way the CHW would communicate among themselves on operational matters, and how the CHW would communicate with the communities and the public health sub-system to which they belong. These differences in the setting where the communications take place lead to narratives that are only understandable or meaningful inside the system where those communications take place or where coupling between the systems is possible.

9.11 Health policy analysis

This section deals with the differentiation between health systems and political systems and policies as written communications. Widely used analytical frameworks address health policies without considering the systemic features of the political and the health systems. Here we cannot give a full account of those frameworks; we give a brief overview of the topic from the Social Systems Theory perspective, considering that the political and health systems are communication-based self-referred, operationally closed systems.

Policies are indeed enacted by the political system, as the maker of *collectively binding* decisions, to be implemented by the other function systems, including the health system. Policies can also be enacted by the health system according to its self-organizing functions. Policies are written communications to orient, set the information scope and channels of communication that implement the policies. Policies that are not thus translated have no real consequences and are irrelevant; therefore policy communications have to be executed as continuous unfolding communications among those concerned.

The political pressures to enact policies may at some point activate the political system. Once activated, the political system discusses, makes decisions, closes the matter, and moves on to other pressing issues, leaving the implementation to the respective systems.[2]

---

2   There is an enormous literature conceptualizing how issues get political attention and go through a decision-making process to eventual policy enactments by a political system. According to Luhmann, the political system is essentially concerned with its own legitimacy, to be continuously confirmed in the decisions it takes. There is

The daily functioning routines of the health systems do not mobilize much interest in the political sphere. Political analysis therefore has to account for the intermittence of political attention, as far as the making of *collectively binding* decisions is at stake, while the life of the health system and its organizations progress at their own pace, determined by their capacities of self-reference and self-reproduction (reproduction of its communications).

On the other hand, health systems and health organizations closely monitor and manage the implementation of the approved policies. It is important to keep in perspective that health policies are intended to have effects in health systems whose largest proportion of resources is continuously dedicated to healthcare services provision with strong inertia and therefore little room for changing established practices. In other words, policies arise in contexts where what is already in place cannot easily change. Rather than having a "blank sheet of paper", health policy-making may have to content itself with "scribbling at the margins", so to speak, narrowing down the ambitions to specific limited programme targets.

Furthermore, as both the political and health systems are based on communications, any change in policies, whether initiated by the health system or by the political system, requires communications that can go back and forth and eventually may become policy texts. The success or failure of policy initiatives may rest on the possibility of eliciting and sustaining such communications.

The article by S. Dalglish et al. (2018), discussing medical power in two case studies of health policymaking in India (on medical specialization) and Niger (on child survival), brings interesting materials for reflections. The authors describe how medical groups, although small and fragmented, exercised policy-making determinant influences by dominating discussions in consultations and conferences and with access to regulatory institutes and committees.

In correspondence to that, the Social Systems Theory would advise researchers to observe the communications and presence/absence of competing

---

a plethora of concepts focusing on structural aspects, diverse range of variables and multiple dynamics trying to give an account of how policies are shaped. However, for the discussion here, the focus is on the theoretical structure by which political decisions taken by the political system become part of the life of the health system and its organizations, as distinct systems differentiated from the political system. We therefore do not delve into the huge contingencies and complexities of policy-making and rather try to fix attention on essential functional and structural aspects of the links between the two systems.

communications that could carry different meanings, presenting self-observations of the system in perhaps convincing terms inside the systems. What needs to be understood are the occurrences of communications and the complexities and specificities involved. Organizations (professional organizations included) that establish communications with other organizations are able to achieve coordination in these processes.

Intentions or interests that are not communicated do not acquire systemic consistency and therefore do not stabilize as communications the systems can recognize. The presumption of power as a position that grants strength and domination to the respective occupiers may distort the observation of policymaking. Communications and power as a communication medium need to be better understood, and power cannot do the work that communication doesn't. The power topic is further discussed in the annex.

The article by G. Walt et al. (2008) presented a picture of the state of affairs of health policy analysis in the international academic literature at the time it was written. Commenting on observations made in reviews of papers on the subject, the authors pointedly indicated that "the main question is often 'what happened', to the neglect of 'what explains what happened'" (Walt et al. 2008, p. 309). This, according to the authors, reflected the lack of or limited use of theoretical frameworks. Theories and frameworks were mainly descriptive rather than explanatory.

From our perspective, the excessive use and dissemination of insufficient frameworks is also responsible for delaying the actual reflection work that needs to be done, putting health policy analysis on firmer theoretical ground. We therefore argue that Luhmann's Social Systems Theory has the elements to reconfigure the debate.

To discuss policy from a Social Systems Theory perspective, we can start with the definition of health policy as adopted in the mentioned article: "It can be useful to think of health policy as embracing 'courses of action (and inaction) that affect the set of institutions, organizations, services and funding arrangements of the health system'" (quoted from Buse et al. 2005, p. 6). Luhmann is emphatic in signalling that *action* does not have the capacity to develop social systems; actions do not require the interlacing with further actions and are thus "weak carriers of meanings".[3]

---

3 "Weak carriers of meaning" is our attempt to put in a few words Luhmann's views expressed for instance in the following words (our translation from Spanish): "a social order is more integrated at the level of attribution of motives than at the

In contrast, communication fulfils all requirements to build social life. Essentially communication requires the enlacement of understandings, linking a communication with past and subsequent ones, permitting the recursive confirmation (or not) of the correct (or not) reception of a communicated meaning. Communication always keeps open the possibility of a "yes" or "no", and therefore is contingent and offers the possibility of selections on both communicating sides.

In comparison, action does not offer a complex enough mean for the development of social life. An action without communication lacks meaning. Only communication can create social life and society. The meaning of an action needs to be communicated to acquire social relevance.

Based on that, we can say that policies are written communications to orient actions and, above all, guide communications, setting information scopes and channels for them. A policy document should be seen as a system communicating and organizing itself. It entails self-references and self-organizing guidance; in other words, it sets the definitions for communications that will then implement the original policy. Policies that are not translated into systems' communicative operations have no real consequences and are thus irrelevant. Illustrating that, policies bring orientations for a system's internal communications on how it should observe and communicate about the policy itself, i.e. the monitoring and evaluation mechanisms.

Policies can originate in the political system as well as in the health system. Once enacted by the political system or by the organizations of the health system (within their scope), and subsequently made operational, a policy becomes integrated into the internal communications of the health system. In that, while becoming operational, the police acquire diverse and often unforeseen complexities that the system will need to deal with. The complexities emerging in the implementation of a policy can go beyond what the policy expected and predicted. The self-observation of the system might identify the excesses of complexities that should be solved. Complexities do not necessarily have unavoidable good or bad meanings; they just arise out of the system/environment relations.

---

level of action itself. Thus, the understanding of motives retrospectively helps to recognize whether an action has occurred" (Luhmann 2005, p. 30). We can add that construction and attribution of motives and objectives can only be made through narrative, i.e. communications, not actions.

The Social System Theory has profound implications for observing health policies, and the genesis of policies in the context of the coupling of two differentiated social systems: the health and the political system. At high level, health policies are, in Luhmann's terms, *collectively binding* decisions taken by the political system to be implemented by the health system and its organizations, which implement them in correspondence to their self-organizing functionalities.

Policies can also be enacted by the public health systems (setting up programmes, for example) or by health organizations (organizing internal services in large complexes of inpatient and outpatient care, for example); these are communications of internal decisions that subsequently have to be executed via communications among those concerned. Regardless of the origin, enacted policies are expected to have effects in health systems' communications.[4]

Policies only become effective when their guidance is communicatively incorporated into the life of the system, and therefore can become part of the system's self-reference and self-reproduction. Only the health system can do the translation of policies' ordinances for itself; such prerogative cannot be delegated or transferred to any external systems.

9.12 Epidemic outbreak

To illustrate how the health system deals with environmental complexities and is then affected by that, we use an example of a simulation of an outbreak of SARS. This example explains that while dealing with complexities the system becomes more complex in the process. In particular, the example also helps to understand the distinction between the system that responds to the outbreak and the outbreak itself. Outbreaks or endemics or epidemics are often mistakenly called systems in modelling and simulation exercises, however they are not systems according to the Social Systems Theory. Outbreaks do not pursue autopoiesis, do not show operational closure and do not use communication as building blocks. Transmission of infectious diseases cannot be understood

---

4   Luhmann's theory about political systems is rich in concepts and cannot be thoroughly explained here. A section in the Annex gives brief explanations about it. For the discussion at this point, it is relevant to signal the theoretical structure by which political decisions taken by the political system become part of the life of the health system and its organizations.

as communications (of meanings) in the sense defined in the Social Systems Theory.

The relevant paper was written by K. Wyss and J. Costa (2003) for the Swiss Federal Office of Public Health, simulating scenarios of a possible outbreak of SARS in Switzerland, considering the impact of possible measures the system could implement. The network of factors and expected health interventions were comprehensively mapped and used for building a stochastic model of the epidemic profile. The modelling allowed the complexity of the outbreak to be taken into account, with its inherent uncertainties, as well as the complexities of the diverse sets of interventions the health system could select from and implement with varied unpredictable rates of successes.

The factors determining the appearance and spread of the disease, considered as environmental factors in the Social System Theory terminology, were addressed as similar to indicators observed in other epidemics. They considered the indicators: arrival of a number of infected individuals; distribution of susceptible population; local transmission by the first cases; incubation period before the onset of the outbreak; population density and distribution of contacts with infected individuals; transmission period; attack rate; case fatality rate; reproductive number R; population and population age and density. Obviously, not all those indicators were included in the models.

On the other side, once the outbreak is detected, the health system would be expected to put in place a number of measures that would include: case detection; contact tracing; quarantine; preventive measures to avoid transmission; isolation of patients; proper disposal of bodies; training of professionals; communication campaigns; acquisition of new drugs and equipment; statistical monitoring; management of responses; and so on. We saw all of that going on in the recent Covid pandemic. The response measures are essentially expected to reduce the rhythm of transmission, disrupting the course of the outbreak. However, the rates of success of each measure and their combined effect are also uncertain and can only be tentatively incorporated in the model as probability functions and intervals.

Based on this rich panorama of factors and interventions, the behaviour of a health system facing an outbreak can be predicted as follows. The health system first recognizes the occurrence of a disease and a possible outbreak in its environment. The system acknowledges that the outbreak is a matter the system has the responsibility to communicate and do something about, and in consequence of that, mobilizes the sets of communications to internally report the events and formulate the decisions to be taken.

There are internal expectations and ready-made (comprehensive or partial) communications to be uttered on specific themes related to risks, contention, monitoring, treatments, etc. elaborated in correspondence to the system's self-produced narratives for explanations and actions related to outbreaks. In a few words, the health system detects the interferences in its domain, makes them the subject of its own concerns, and deploys the relevant communications.

Different health systems may differ in relation to the capacity to identify an outbreak and the type, rapidity, intensity, extension, etc. of their response. The differences might be linked to relevant internal characteristics of the system and its self-defined ways of tackling outbreaks, as the system understands it. Once a system sets its response in motion, a chain of recurrent communications are then recurrently reproduced and maintained. The outbreak then becomes what the system and those working alongside it say about it.

The health system has to construct an internal narrative explaining (to itself in the first instance) what the outbreak is about and the peculiar characteristics to be tackled by measures the system will then put in place. The system needs to take account of all the fields of intervention where it will need to deploy its resources. It goes through a process of internal differentiation with new sets of communications and respective operations and addressees (the locus of new responsibilities) becoming functional.

The scenario can be depicted as follows. Sections of the health system will be handling treatment guidelines and isolation rules to treat the sick. Some divisions will deal with social communication and communication to professionals inside and outside the system. Other sections will take care of the logistics of tracing contacts and assuring they will be properly quarantined for the necessary time. Others still will be dealing with the monitoring and statistics of the outbreak. Other actors will carry out procurement of emergency materials, medicines and all that is required to treat patients, quarantine contacts, as well as deliver prophylaxis. Still, another team will carry out political and decision-making activities, exchanging communications with other systems to be made aware of the outbreak and perform activities within their scope of competences. Each of the created divisions and sections will need to put in motion their own rules of functioning and engagement.

In short, the overall mobilization shows the health system becoming more complex, generating a range of additional internal communication with new semantics. If the system is for the first time dealing with a large outbreak, after it subsides the system will display features that it did not have previously. It will acquire operational competences and the knowledge/communications required to deploy those competences. The complexity of the epidemic will have been translated into control measures, increasing the complexity of the health system, and having long-lasting effects.

In Luhmann's words: "Only complexity can reduce complexity" (Luhmann 1995, p. 26). Only the complexity of the system can reduce the complexity of the environment. The restructuring of competences and responsibilities taking place inside the health system is how the complexity of an outbreak is tackled. The aim should not be to reduce environmental complexity or to turn it into simplicity; this would not be possible. Instead, the system should "embrace" complexity, so to speak. A more complex division of labour, new communication channels, revised assignment of responsibilities, reviewed distribution of resources and skills are, for example, aspects that might change irreversibly once the autopoiesis of the health system leads it to another level of response.

Acknowledging that by tackling an outbreak a health system will become more complex, and will change the sets and conditions of the communications it sustains, should have significant bearing on devising the strategies the system needs to adopt. This understanding also raises important considerations for any initiative aiming at strengthening health systems.

Final Remarks – Science or Technology

In this last chapter of the book attention is on the use of theories in academic and business contexts. Let's take the distinction between science and technology, with the second understood as translation of the first, with the purpose of bringing about improvements of some sort. The distinction is clear for the separation of, for instance, manufacturers making new designs of cars without having to review or reconceptualize any of the scientific knowledge about metallurgy, electric and electronic circuits, mechanical engineering, aerodynamics, and so on. Making pieces, tools and objects that are advantageous regarding efficiency, aesthetics, ergonomics and other parameters of judgement, rarely requires new scientific theories or hypotheses. This is what technology is about.

By the same token, we can comfortably say that most of what has been published in the field of health system, health systems thinking or health systems strengthening can be classified as technology. In this case, the manufacturers are in the academy, providing new designs to go into the testing grounds of the health systems of the world. Very little science is actually produced; most works consist in redesigning what has already been established in scientific fields or are still tentative drafts.

Were each advance in the car manufacturing industry to be described and published in the literature, there would possibly be as many articles on the subject as are found in the health systems literature. But there is no interest in such publications, because at the end of the day the selling of the final product in the car market is all that matters.

On the health systems literature, on the other hand, the market for such final products is limited to a small set of sponsors in the international arena, in search of technical advice and willing to pay for health strengthening initiatives in countries supposedly in need of them. In fact, besides the technical advice, the main products in this industry, the publications themselves, around which much of academic life revolves, are to a large extent what are at stake.

The industry of producing such technologies, health systems thinking for instance, is less concerned with making changes in the real world – like fancy new cars speeding along the highways of the world – but rather with generating publishable articles to reach high scores in the citation indexes of academic journals, or influential positions in the agenda-making of research and advising sponsors. If we abstract the nature of the products, we see that we are dealing with the same thing, namely technological innovations. The published health systems technology sustains both the related advice and academic careers in the respective industries.

It is easy to identify technological initiatives because they come as a result of fixing attention on a few features for improvement. What is relevant is to adequately justify the techniques of the interventions, and that new design with new potentially successful buzzwords is brought to the "market". In-depth scientific exploration is not required, as airplane designers would very well agree while considering different designs for the fitting of the interior of the cabins; all that they are concerned about are techniques for manufacture and testing to adjust the designs.

For technological initiatives, no deep discussion of the logic, validity and precision of concepts are needed. Simple, reasonably measurable definitions are enough. Resilience, community participation, empowerment and ownership are just a few of those terms that are used in academic health systems communications, giving an impression of fair understanding, nevertheless leaving crucial problems unaddressed.

For instance, what is the nature of power or empowerment? What are the limits and qualification basis of resilience? Is negative resilience, keeping bad habits in place, as relevant as the positive one? To what extent does participation inhibit or prevent participation? How and what is actually possible to own when ownership is intended? In these kinds of questions, not only techniques are matters of concerns; the very nature of the phenomenon, the concepts expressing them and the possibility of observing them are of central interest.

But, as interior designers of airplanes would reject as unnecessary any discussion about the theories of molecular structures of matter explaining why plastic of certain density is amenable to taking on shapes for the fitting panels, those aiming at publishing articles in academic journals would not get deeper into reflections about the meanings of resilience, power, participation, etc. They already know the technology "market" they are in, and it does not require such exhaustive exercises. A successful term in this market is the one that produces echoes throughout a number of publications and does not quickly exhaust its attractive potential, no matter how superficial and fragile it still is.

We can here open a brief parenthesis and talk about the art social system, also a system to which Luhmann dedicated his attention.[1] Art techniques of painting, sculpting, playing music, etc. may generate products that are appreciated but are not recognized as art. The art system itself does not recognize them as art because they do not fulfil criteria of novelty, originality, singularity, surprise, innovation, breaking with established traditions, and other standards of judgement the art system creates for itself. Likewise, technological application and replication can be easily multiplied. But scientific advances require novelties and incursions into what is not already known, not just simple repetition of the techniques already established.

However, it must be said that in the medical science field, the enormous amount of technical publications that can also be considered technology nevertheless have specific relevance. The publication of collections of evidence from results of treatments, clinical trials, review of publications, etc. does not need to represent breakthroughs or new theoretical approaches in their specific field. Most publications simply report on the results of application of exams or therapeutic techniques, and do not propose or suggest any new theoretical view on the studied phenomenon. Nevertheless, the reported evidence helps other professionals to find possible solutions for treating patients with similar problems. This is undoubtedly of high relevance for the development of medical science and the theoretical work that can use those observations.

In the field of health systems, on the other hand, where the theoretical base is very fragile or even non-existent, the collection of lots of evidence does not contribute in the same way that medical techniques evidence does. This contrast is partially due to the fact that medical science has a solid theoretical/empirical basis (in areas such as pharmacology, physiology, biochemistry, pathology, radiology, surgery, and so on), while health systems are at the first stage of technical development, using all sorts of references from external fields (sociology, epidemiology, psychology, economics, management, political science, cybernetics, and so on), trying to find its identity.

---

1 If interested, the reader can dive into Luhmann's (2000) book *Art as a Social System*, with a deep and thorough analysis of the evolution of the art system to its current stage as seen in contemporary artworks, museums and galleries.

In correspondence to that, all technological approaches to health systems are tentative; the maxim "one size does not fit all" is often reminded as the diversity of variables involved and the peculiarities of each context continue to multiply. The health system "boat" seems to be lost in a storm of unending new factors and variables, sailing through it with the "thinking" option, which does not seem to reveal the limiting horizons and coordinates to navigate a vast, endless sea.

The researchers may take a health system topic as a subject – for instance, reference and counter-reference from primary healthcare to secondary healthcare facilities – and then go to the field to observe and take measurements. Each new context of study will offer plenty of new variables to take into account for the judgements of what seems to work or doesn't. As opposed to the medical researchers with their sets of well-established theoretical references, the health system researchers will have to look for ad hoc references used by other empirical works or borrow some from other fields of knowledge; they will have to move on and be happy with that. Then, they will go out into the field, make observations, narrate what was observed and that is it; no theory is confirmed or discarded, or even mentioned. Often, there are no theories to talk about, and the work would not have the ambition to contribute to the development or refinement of theoretical knowledge; and yet very little is added as evidence for technical intervention designs, given the plethora of variables, diversity and specificity of any social context.

The publication may just say that in countries "X", "Y" and "Z", x %, y % and z % of PHC patients are referred to secondary level, and some factors explaining the differences are listed; no theoretical base is needed. This is obviously technology trying to figure out the best "fit", not science. In this, the researcher may be easy prey to ideological currents that may imperceptibly influence the selection of variables. Ideology is effective in occupying spaces left unattended in theoretical fields.

Yes, we do have to admit and give credit to the usefulness of narrative description of contextualized experience. Someone may get suggestions from those narratives, and be inspired by them for the work they may have to organize in another setting. The value of the testing of tools and collection of empirical data should not be disregarded. We are not advocating that it should be ignored. However, attention needs to be given to theoretical work per se.

The hard work of theoretical construction does not promise simple success. A polemic and difficult conceptual body may not attract much attention, particularly from those looking for quick fixes and piecemeal approaches that can speedily be translated into a new generation of technological products, meaning publishable new articles, even if using half-baked concepts. It does not matter if reality artificially narrowed down at the site of observations is constructed by discarding crucial elements. The technology "market" is sovereign within its domain. The demand for technologies is not the same as the demand for scientific knowledge. The "market" for health systems technologies is well developed in the academic and development-aid industry worlds, on the other hand, the "market" for health systems theory has still to emerge.

For the Social Systems Theory, science is a functional system operating with communications based on true/false binary code in connection with theories and corresponding evidence search techniques. Technology is not a function system; it rather comprehends normalized, standardized communications inside any function system and, more specifically, communications concerning applications and whether they work or not. Luhmann (2007, p. 416) has an interesting formulation for the problem of technique: "the technique .. operates orthogonally in relation to the operational closure of the autopoietic systems", thus assuring structural coupling between *function systems* and their environment. In other words, any function system can incorporate technical communications (and relevant technologies) for their specific matters of concern. In this sense, the science function system may incorporate techniques for its considerations in distinguishing true and false, but it is not concerned with the usefulness of techniques, which may or may not be absorbed by other function systems for their own sake.

To this discussion we may add a comment on the low relevance given to exclusively theoretical papers. With rare exceptions of specific journals, most academic journals require empirical data analysis, and reject papers without that. But they are not demanding on the theories employed, never mind the quality of the concepts deployed for fieldwork observations. Perhaps it is necessary to advocate for better theoretical scrutiny of concepts deployed in empirical studies, and the acceptance of strictly theoretical reflection on conceptual frameworks used without any consideration of consistency and adequacy.

Final comment

Addressing health systems as social systems requires a notion of system different from what has been used in health systems studies. This new way of speaking will certainly find resistance as the word "system" has been used for decades without a precise definition. It will not be easy to convince users accustomed to the previous uses, of the value of a new semantic with the same sign (the word system). We may talk of "conceptual resilience" here. It is unlikely that the new concepts succeed in bringing about widespread acceptance and recognition, particularly when they sound complicated and counter-intuitive in relation to settled notions.

Yes, health systems have been talked and written about over the last decades in many international and academic forums. Many operations, investment and initiatives communicate and try to make health systems across the world into visible functioning organizations that can deliver what is expected of them, with collected knowledge and resources. The success of a call for better understanding of the working of those huge on-going apparatuses is not certain.

The term "health system" has opened a world of associations. Anyone engaged in any health system knows is communicating within a comprehensive whole called health system. The institutions, organizations, services and personnel are all part of this constructed conceptual whole, using the semantics that make the universe of communications of a health system. The self-reference does not need to recognize that it is what it is in any particular or rigorously defined sense; self-reference advances even with contingent forms.

So, the terms "health system as a social system" may become well understood and incorporated into the communications of the science system, but may take longer to become normal "currency" in the pragmatic, operations-orientated health systems. Furthermore, a new paradigm of observation is required; as opposed to the unilateral medical observation of the human body, the observation of social systems is observation of observers observing observers.

References

The consulted literature is listed in this chapter. It includes Luhmann's books in English and Spanish translations. Besides that, several relevant texts, written by those who studied Luhmann's theory, as well as those who Luhmann mentioned and borrowed concepts from, are included here. Furthermore, the publications from where the cases, studies and health systems thinking definitions and tools have been used are also included in these references. The references are organized in two sections, one with articles and reports, and the other with books and book chapters.

Articles and reports

Abiiro G. and De Allegri M. – "Universal health coverage from multiple perspectives: a synthesis of conceptual literature and global debates", *BMC International Health and Human Rights* (2015) 15:17

Adam T. and de Savigny D. – "Systems thinking for strengthening health systems in LMICs: need for a paradigm shift", *Health Policy and Planning* 2012; 27:iv1–iv3

An J. – "Social networks and health: models, methods, and applications, Health Informatics Research", 2012 December; 18(4) 287–289 (Book review)

Atun R. – "Health systems, systems thinking and innovation", *Health Policy and Planning* 2012; 27:iv4–iv8

Azline A. et al. – "Policy arena of health policy-making process in developing countries", *International Journal of Public Health and Clinical Sciences*: 2289–7577. Vol. 5: No. 3, 2018

Balabanova, D., McKee, M., Mills, A., Walt, G., Haines, A. – "What can global health institutions do to help strengthen health systems in low-income countries?" *Health Research Policy and Systems* 2010

Barasa E., Cloete K. and Gilson L. – "From bouncing back, to nurturing emergence: reframing the concept of resilience in health systems strengthening", *Health Policy Plan*. 2017 November 01; 32(Suppl. 3)

Bennett, S., Frenk, J., Mills, A., – "The evolution of the field of Health Policy and Systems Research and outstanding challenges", *Health Research Policy and Systems* (2018)

Blanchet K. – "How to Facilitate Social Contagion?" *International Journal of Health Policy and Management*, 2013, 1(3), 189–192

Blanchet K., Nam S., Ramalingam B. and Pozo-Martin F. – "Governance and Capacity to Manage Resilience of Health Systems: Towards a New Conceptual Framework", *Int. J Health Policy Management*. 2017, 6(8), 431–435

Bommes, M. and Tacke, V. – "Luhmann's Systems Theory and Network Theory", Chapter 13 in *Niklas Luhmann and Organization Studies*, edited by Seidl, D. and Becker, K., CBS Press, 2006, Denmark.

Brainard J. and Hunter P. – "Do complexity-informed health interventions work? A scoping review", *Implementation Science* (2016) 11:127

Brans M. and Rossbach S. – "The autopoiesis of administrative systems: Niklas Luhmann on public administration and public policy", *Public Administration* Vol. 75, 1997 (417–439)

Carey G. et al. – "Systems science and systems thinking for public health: a systematic review of the field", *BMJ Open* 2015; 5:e009002

Chughtai S. and Blanchet K. – "Systems thinking in public health: a bibliographic contribution to a meta-narrative review", *Health Policy and Planning*, 32, 2017, 585–594

Dalglish, S., Sriram, V., Scott, K. and Rodríguez, D. – "A framework for medical power in two case studies of health policymaking in India and Niger", *Global Public Health*, pages 542–554 | Published online 2018

de Savigny D. et al. – "Introducing vouchers for malaria prevention in Ghana and Tanzania: context and adoption of innovation in health systems", *Health Policy and Planning*, Volume 27, Issue suppl_4, October 2012, Pages iv32–iv43

Ensor T. – "Informal payments for health care in transition economies", *Social Science & Medicine* 58 (2004) 237–246

Eriksen T., Kerry R., Mumford S., Lie S. and Anjum R. – "At the borders of medical reasoning: aetiological and ontological challenges of medically unexplained symptoms", *Philosophy, Ethics, and Humanities in Medicine* 2013, 8:11

Fana V. Feng-Jen J. Tsaic C. Branden N. Nabil V. Scott W. – "Dedicated health systems strengthening of the Global Fund to Fight AIDS, Tuberculosis, and Malaria: an analysis of grants", *Int. Health* 2017; 9: 50–57

Galichet B. et al. – "Linking programmes and systems: lessons from the GAVI Health Systems Strengthening window", *Tropical Medicine and International Health* volume 15 no 2 pp. 208–215 February 2010

Gautier L., De Allegri M. and Ridde V. – "How is the discourse of performance-based financing shaped at the global level? A post-structural analysis", *Globalization and Health* (2019) 15:6

Goldberg J. and Bryant M. – "Country ownership and capacity building: the next buzzwords in health systems strengthening or a truly new approach to development?" *BMC Public Health* 2012, 12:531

Gore R. and Parker R. – "Analyzing power and politics in health policies and systems", *Global Public Health* 2019, vol. 14, no. 4, 481–488

Günther, G. – "Life as Poly-Contexturality", Vordenker 2004 (Paper)

Hafner T. and Shiffman J. – "The emergence of global attention to health systems strengthening", *Health Policy and Planning* 2013; 28:41–50

Harris P. et al. – "A glossary of theories for understanding power and policy for health equity", *J Epidemiology and Community Health* 2020; 0:1–5

Homer J. and Hirsch G. – "System Dynamics Modeling for Public Health: Background and Opportunities", *Am J Public Health*. 2006; 96 (vol. 3), 19–25

Husain L. – "Policy experimentation and innovation as a response to complexity in China's management of health reforms", *Globalization and Health* (2017) 13:54

Jenkins C., Hien H., Chi B. and Santin O. – "What works in global health partnerships? Reflections on a collaboration between researchers from Vietnam and Northern Ireland", *BMJ Global Health* 2021; 6:e005535

Joseph, S. – "Impact Assessment of Accreditation in Primary and Secondary Public Health-care Institutions in Kerala, India", *Indian J Public Health* 2021; 65:110-5

Kim H. – "The implicit ideological function of the global health field and its role in maintaining relations of power", *BMJ Global Health* 2021; 6:e005620

King M. and Schütz M. – "The Ambitious Modesty of Niklas Luhmann" *Journal of Law and Society*, Sep., 1994, Vol. 21, No. 3 (Sep., 1994), pp. 261–287

Kroeger F. – "Facework: creating trust in systems, institutions and organizations", *Cambridge Journal of Economics* 2017, 41, 487–514

Kroeger F. – "Unlocking the treasure trove: How can Luhmann's Theory of Trust enrich trust research?" *Journal of Trust Research*, 2019, vol. 9, no. 1, 110–124

Kutzin J. – "Health financing for universal coverage and health system performance: concepts and implications for policy", *Bull World Health Organ 2013;* 91: 602–611

Kutzin J. and Sparkes S. – "Health systems strengthening, universal health coverage, health security and resilience", *Bull World Health Organ* 2016; 94:2

Leegwater A., Wong W. and Avila C. – "A concise, health service coverage index for monitoring progress towards universal health coverage", *BMC Health Services Research* (2015) 15:230

Luhmann N. and Fuchs S. – "Tautology and Paradox in the Self-Descriptions of Modern Society", *Sociological Theory*, Vol. 6, No. 1 (Spring, 1988), pp. 21–37

Mills, A., Gilson, L., Hanson, K., Palmer, N., Lagarde, M. – "What do we mean by rigorous health-systems research?", *The Lancet* Vol. 372, 1527–1529, November 1, 2008

Mirzoev T. and Kane S. – "What is health systems responsiveness? Review of existing knowledge and proposed conceptual framework", *BMJ Glob Health* 2017;2:e000486

Mol A. and Law J. – "Regions, Networks and Fluids: Anaemia and Social Topology", *Social Studies of Science*, Vol. 24, No. 4 (Nov., 1994), pp. 641–671

Munir K. and Worm I. – "Health systems strengthening in German development cooperation: making the case for a comprehensive strategy", *Globalization and Health* (2016) 12:81

Paina, L., Bennett, S., Ssengooba, F. and Peters, D. – "Advancing the application of systems thinking in health: exploring dual practice and its management in Kampala, Uganda", *Health Research Policy and Systems* 2014, 12:41

Rhodes M. – "A network based theory of health systems and cycles of well-being", *International Journal of Health Policy and Management*, 2013, 1(1), 7–15

Rizvi S., Douglas R., Williams O. and Hill P. – "The political economy of universal health coverage: a systematic narrative review", *Health Policy and Planning*, 35, 2020, 364–372

Sabot K., Wickremasinghe D., Blanchet K., Avan B. and Schellenberg J. – "Use of social network analysis methods to study professional advice and performance among healthcare providers: a systematic review", *Systematic Reviews* (2017) 6:208

Scott K., George A. and Ved R. – "Taking stock of 10 years of published research on the ASHA programme: examining India's national community health worker programme from a health systems perspective", *Health Research Policy and Systems* (2019) 17:29

Seidl D. – "Luhmann's theory of autopoietic social systems", Ludwig-Maximilians-Universität München, Munich School of Management. 2004

Seidl D. and Becker K. – "Organizations as Distinction Systems", Sage pub 2006, Volume 13(1): 9–35

Shakarishvili, G. et al. – "Health systems strengthening: a common classification and framework for investment analysis", *Health Policy and Planning* 2011; 26:316–326

Sriram V. et al. – "10 best resources on power in health policy and systems in low- and middle-income countries", *Health Policy and Planning*, 2018, 1–11

Stepurko T, Pavlova M, Gryga I, Murauskiene L and Groot W. – "Informal payments for health care services: The case of Lithuania, Poland and Ukraine", *Journal of Eurasian Studies* 6 (2015) 46 – 58

Swanson R. et al. – "Rethinking health systems strengthening: key systems thinking tools and strategies for transformational change", *Health Policy and Planning* 2012; 27:iv54–iv61

Swanson R. et al. – "Toward a Consensus on Guiding Principles for Health Systems Strengthening", *PLoS Medicine*, December 2010 | Volume 7 | Issue 12

The Global Fund – "Advisory Paper on Resilient and Sustainable Systems for Health, Technical Review Panel", Geneva, The Global Fund, October 2021

Tichenor M. and Sridhar D. – "Universal health coverage, health systems strengthening, and the World Bank", *BMJ* 2017; 358:j3347

USAID – "Global Health Initiative (GHI) Principle Paper – Health Systems Strengthening", The US Government 2012

Valentinov V, Roth S. and Will M. – "Stakeholder Theory: A Luhmannian Perspective", *Administration & Society* 2019, Vol. 51(5) 826–849

Varela F., Maturana H. and Uribe R. – "Autopoiesis: The Organization of Living Systems, its Characterization and a Model". *Biosystems* 1974 5:187-96

Vassell A. and Nguyen T. – "Theories of Social Systems: Implications for Health Care System", *International Journal of Psychological Studies* Vol. 4, No. 2; June 2012

Walt, G. et al. – "'Doing' health policy analysis: methodological and conceptual reflections and challenges", *Health Policy and Planning* 2008; 23:308–317

Wyss K. and Costa J. – "Assessment of the costs of a SARS epidemic in Switzerland", a study for the Swiss Federal Office of Public Health, 2003 (Study report)

Books and book chapters

Ahlemeyer, H. (2001) – "Management by Complexity: Redundancy and Variety in Organizations", chapter 3 in *Sociocybernetics: Complexity, Autopoiesis and Observation of Social Systems*, edited by Geyer, F. and van der Zouwen, J., ed. Greenwood Press, London

Baecker, D. (2006) – "The Design of Organization in Society", chapter 9 in *Niklas Luhmann and Organization Studies*, edited by Seidl, D. and Helge, K., ed. Liber and Copenhagen Business School Press, Frederiksberg C.

Bakken, T. and Hernes, T. (editors) (2003) – *Autopoietic Organization Theory, Drawing on Niklas Luhmann's Social Systems Perspective*, ed. Copenhagen Business School Press, Copenhagen.

Blanchet, K. and Shearer, J. (2017) – "Network analysis: a tool for understanding social network behaviour of a system", chapter 7 in *Applied Systems Thinking for Health Systems Research, a methodological handbook*, edited by de Savigny et al., Open University Press

Borch, C. (2011) – *Niklas Luhmann, key sociologists*, ed. Routledge, New York

Buse K., Mays N. and Walt G. – *Making Health Policy*, Open University Press, McGraw-Hill Education, England, 2005

Bynum, W. (2008) – *The History of Medicine: a very short introduction*, Oxford University Press, New York

Canguilhem, G. (1978) – *On the Normal and the Pathological*, ed. D. Reidel Publishing Company, London

De Savigny, D., Blanchet, K. and Adam, T. (2017) – *Applied Systems Thinking for Health Systems Research, a methodological handbook*, Open University Press, London

Drepper, T. (2006) – "Organization and Society", chapter 8 in *Niklas Luhmann and Organization Studies*, edited by Seidl, D. and Helge, K., ed. Liber and Copenhagen Business School Press, Frederiksberg C.

Foerster, H. (2014) – *The Beginning of Heaven and Earth Has no Name: Seven Days with Second-Order Cybernetics*, ed. Fordham University Press, California

Foucault, M. (2003) – *The Birth of the Clinic, an archaeology of medical perception*, ed. Routledge, London

Friedman, B. (2008) – "Policy Analysis as Organizational Analysis", chapter 23 in *The Oxford Handbook of Public Policy*, edited by Moran, M, Rein, M. and Goodin, R., Oxford University Press, Oxford

Habermas, J. (2007) – "Excursus on Luhmann's appropriation of the Philosophy of the Subject through Systems Theory", chapter 12 in *The Philosophical Discourse of Modernity: twelve lectures*, Polity Press, UK

Harman, G. (2018) – *Object-Oriented Ontology – a new theory of everything*, ed Pelican Books,

Johnson, N. (2011) – *Simply complexity, a clear guide to Complexity Theory*, ed. Oneworld Publications, Oxford

King, M. and Thornhill, C. (2003) – *Niklas Luhmann's Theory of Politics and Law*, ed. Palgrave, New York

Knudsen, M. (2012) – "Structural coupling between organizations and function systems: looking at standards in health care", chapter 5 in *The Illusion of Management Control, A Systems Theoretical Approach to Managerial Technologies*, edited by Thygesen, N., ed. Palgrave, London

Knudsen, M. and Vogd, W. (editors) (2015) – *Systems Theory and the Sociology of Health and Illness, Observing healthcare*, ed. Routledge, New York

Latour, B., Harman, G. and Erdélyi, P. (2011) – *The Prince and the Wolf. Latour and Harman at the LSE*, Zero Books, John Hunt Publishing,

Law, J. and Hassard, J. (2005) – *Actor Network Theory and after*, Blackwell Publishing, Oxford

Laws, D. and Hajer, M. (2008) – "Policy in Practice", chapter 19 in *The Oxford Handbook of Public Policy*, edited by Moran, M, Rein, M. and Goodin, R., Oxford University Press, Oxford

Leydesdorff, L. (2002) – *Communicative competencies and the structuration of expectations: the creative tension between Habermas' critical theory and Luhmann's social systems theory*, University of Amsterdam

Luhmann, N. (1990) – *Essays on Self-Reference*, Columbia University Press, New York

Luhmann, N. (1990) – *Political Theory in the Welfare State*, ed. Walter de Gruyter, Berlin

Luhmann, N. (1995) – *Social Systems*, ed. Stanford University Press, Stanford

Luhmann, N. (1998) – *Complejidad y Modernidad, de la unidad a la diferencia*, Ed. Trotta, Madrid

Luhmann, N. (2000) – *Art as a Social System*, Stanford University Press, Stanford

Luhmann, N. (2002) – *Theories of Distinction, re-describing the description of modernity*, Stanford University Press, Stanford

Luhmann, N. (2005) – *Poder*, Anthropos Editorial, Barcelona

Luhmann, N. (2007a) – *La Sociedad de la Sociedad*, ed. Herder, Cuidad de México

Luhmann, N. (2007b) – *The Reality of the Mass Media*, Polity Press, Cambridge

Luhmann, N. (2008) – *Law as a Social System*, Oxford University Press, Oxford
Luhmann, N. (2013) – *Introduction to Systems Theory*, ed. Polity Press, Cambridge
Luhmann, N. (2014) – *Sociología Política*, ed. Trotta, Madrid
Luhmann, N. (2015) – *Sociedad y sistema: la ambición de la teoría*, ed. Paidós, Barcelona
Luhmann, N. (2016) – "El código de la medicina", chapter 6 in *Distinciones directrices*, ed. Centro de Investigaciones Sociológicas (CIS), Madrid
Luhmann, N. (2017a) – *La Economía de la Sociedad*, ed. Herder, Cuidad de México
Luhmann, N. (2017b) – *Trust and Power*, ed. Polity Press, Cambridge
Luhmann, N. (2018) – *Organization and Decision*, ed. Cambridge University Press, Cambridge
Luhmann, N. (2018) – *The New Boss*, ed. Polity Press, Cambridge
Meyer, S., Gibson, B. and Ward, P. (2015) – "Niklas Luhmann: Social Systems Theory and the Translation of Public Health Research", chapter 22 in *The Palgrave Handbook of Social Theory in Health, Illness and Medicine*, edited by Collyer, F., ed. Palgrave, New York
Moeller, Hans-Georg (2005) – *Luhmann Explained: From Souls to Systems*, ed. Open Court, Chicago
Moeller, Hans-Georg (2012) – *The Radical Luhmann*, ed. Columbia University Press, New York
Mol, A. (2002) a – *The body multiple, ontology in medical practice*, ed. Duke University Press
Mol, A. (2002) b – "Cutting Surgeons, Walking Patients: Some Complexities Involved in Comparing", in *Complexities, Social Studies of Knowledge Practices*, edited by John Law and Annemarie Mol, ed. Duke University Press
Muñoz, D and de Savigny, D. (2017) – "Processing mapping: a tool for visualizing system processes from end-to-end", chapter 9 in *Applied Systems Thinking for Health Systems Research, a methodological handbook*, edited by De Savigny, D., Blanchet, K. and Adam, T., Open University Press, London
Olivier, J. et al. (2017) – "Systems approaches in health systems research: approaches for embedding research", chapter 2 in *Applied Systems Thinking for Health Systems Research, a methodological handbook*, edited by De Savigny, D., Blanchet, K. and Adam, T., Open University Press, London
Parsons, T. (1954) – *Essays in Sociological Theory*, The Free Press, New York
Rasch, W. (2000) – *Niklas Luhmann's Modernity, The Paradoxes of Differentiation*, ed. Stanford University Press, Stanford
Reynolds, M. and Wilding, H. (2017) – "Boundary critique: an approach for framing methodological design", chapter 3 in *Applied Systems Thinking for*

Health Systems Research, a methodological handbook, edited by De Savigny, D., Blanchet, K. and Adam, T., Open University Press, London

Seidl, D. (2006) – "The Basic Concepts of Luhmann's Theory of Social Systems" chapter 1 in *Niklas Luhmann and Organization Studies*, edited by Seidl, D. and Helge, K., ed. Liber and Copenhagen Business School Press, Frederiksberg C.

Seidl, D. and Becker, K. (2006) – *Niklas Luhmann and Organization Studies*, edited by Seidl, D. and Becker, K., ed Liber and Copenhagen Business School Press, Frederiksberg C.

Seidl, D. and Mormann, H. (2014) – "Nicklas Luhmann as Organization Theorist", chapter 7 in *The Oxford Handbook of Sociology, Social Theory and Organization Studies*, edited by Adler, P. Du Gay, P., Morgan, G. and Reed, M., ed. Oxford University Press, New York

Spencer-Brown, G. (2015) – *Laws of Form*, ed. Bohmeier Verlag, Leipzig

Tomaia-Cotsel, A. et al. (2017) – "Causal loop diagrams: a tool for visualizing emergent system behaviour", chapter 6 in *Applied Systems Thinking for Health Systems Research, a methodological handbook*, edited by De Savigny, D., Blanchet, K. and Adam, T., Open University Press, London

Vogd, W. (2015) – "Arranging medical and economic logics: investigating the influence of economic controlling in an internal medicine department", chapter 5, in *Systems Theory and the Sociology of Health and Illness Observing Healthcare*, ed. by Knudsen, M. and Vogd, W., Routledge

World Health Organization (2007) – *Everybody's Business: Strengthening Health Systems to Improve Health Outcomes: WHO's Framework for Action*, WHO Geneva

World Health Organization (2009) – *Systems thinking for health systems strengthening*, edited by Don de Savigny and Taghreed Adam, WHO Geneva

World Health Organization (2010) – *Monitoring the building blocks of health systems: a Handbook of indicators and their measurement strategies*, WHO Geneva

World Health Organization (2017) – *World Report on Health Policy and Systems Research*, WHO Geneva

Annex – Advanced Topics

Additional concepts of the theory and a few complementary definitions of concepts already presented are discussed in this Annex. Due to their complex formulation, they are included here, making the main text of the book as easy to read as possible, avoiding overwhelming the reader who is encountering Luhmann's work for the first time. This Annex also offers a brief description of Luhmann's theoretical formulations about power and the political system.

A.1 Additional concepts

Paradoxes and removal of paradoxes

In Luhmann's terms, all distinctions are paradoxical for being a unit of a difference. Dealing with distinctions and corresponding observations and communications, the systems need to remove paradoxes from the distinctions, which means following processes to remove their paradoxical nature, focusing on only one side of the distinction at a time, without attending to the necessary contrasting notions of the opposite side. The systems employ many strategies to that purpose, such as using decisions previously made as justification for new decisions. Paradoxes carry the risk of preventing determinability and the loss of connection between operations (communications), therefore one side needs to be privileged, and previous decisions offer that possibility. For instance, in dealing with the challenge of allergies and autoimmune diseases, the provision of care needs to stick to the sickness side and remove the indeterminacy of considering that the body is having a normal reaction although against mistaken factors or disproportionately. The symptoms of sickness therefore have to be treated. Iatrogenic psychiatric diseases, with aggravation of symptoms over the course of a hospital admission, may be considered another of such example. Systems' self-reference is also an example of where paradoxes must be avoided (see below the paragraph on self-reference).

Decision, decision paradox, uncertainty absorption and decision premises

Decisions are the main feature in organizations' operations. But decisions are paradoxical in two respects: either when the chosen option is evidently the best and therefore there is no decision to be made, or when the alternatives have equal values and uncertainties and therefore a decision cannot be made. However, decisions are indeed taken and for that a process of *removing paradoxes* (see above) needs to happen. Luhmann says that a decision only becomes a decision as such when a subsequent decision is taken to implement it. In this line of thought, a decision connects to another and subsequent ones in such a way that those making the decisions do not need to go back to the basis and evidence of the previous decisions; thus, decisions become *premises* for those that follow. This connectivity *absorbs uncertainties*, removes the paradox from attention, as the new decisions do not need to address the uncertainties concerning the previous ones when they were made. Luhmann identifies three types of *decision premises: programmes, communication channels* and *personnel*. Earlier decisions incorporated into programmes, personnel and communication channels absolve uncertainties and create the grounds for making decisions by removing the need for argumentation about whether a decision being considered is appropriate or not. A decision is then made on the basis of previous ones that are mentioned as part of the justification. Furthermore, in his late writings, Luhmann introduced another type of decision premise, *undecided decisions*, which characterize decisions that have never been the object of explicit decision processes. He identified two types: *organizational culture* and *cognitive routines*.

Re-entering

Re-entering happens when a distinction enters one of its sides; as, for instance, when a system produces internally an image of the environment (always partial) from which it distinguishes itself through the system/environment's founding distinction. On the system side of the system/environment distinction, the system can present a representation of the distinction itself.

Medium and form

Mediums can only be observed through the forms they take. Forms can only appear if there is a medium to make it possible. Forms present tight connections between the elements that compose them, while the connections are loose in a medium. Medium and forms are essential for communications in any social system. Luhmann speaks about the medium of law, the medium of power, and others.

Symbolically generalized medium of communication

This is perhaps one of the most difficult topics in the theory. Luhmann identifies a number of mediums of communication that are of central relevance as symbols linking motivations and selections in the differentiated function systems. For instance, he mentions the symbolically generalized medium of communication (SGMC) of power, money, law, love, art and truth, among others, providing pervasive reference in the respective systems, facilitating specifications and acceptance of communications. The SGMC increases the chances of accepting communications that otherwise would be highly improbable. For instance, the SGMC of power increases the acceptability of decisions enacted and respective messages emanating from those holding positions of power. In the health system, all involved in healthcare provision know that what is at stake is the distinction between health and sickness and all the communications are accepted as referring to the sickness side. In this sense, we can say that health is a SGMC.

Contingency

Formally speaking, in Luhmann's texts, contingency refers to the condition whereby something is neither necessary nor impossible, and could be different. The term appears constantly in his texts, with relevant implications in relation to observations, selections, communications and decisions, which, in being contingent, can always be different.

Formula of contingency

This concept refers to the function system's specific means of adopting symbolic references that although never fully explained are of high practical importance. For instance, the notion of justice can never play a role in a decision of the legal system, which characterizes the legality or illegality of the act being adjudicated when making its decisions. The expectation is that justice is upheld in all judgements, without having normative power over them. Justice is the achieved outcome of consistent application of the law in all adjudicated cases. Formulas of contingencies are used for rhetorical justification, as for instance the term "cure" can be used in the health system's communications as an overall claim of the objective of all medical actions.

Meaning

In Luhmann's formal definition, meaning is the unit of the difference between a selection and the other possibilities. In other words, the medium of meaning allows the creation of forms that differentiate between actuality and potentiality. The meaning of a word is the selection of an actual possibility vis-à-vis the others that remain potential for not being selected.

Complexity and complexity reduction

A formal definition says that complexity is the condition of having too many elements and relations so that the elements cannot be related to all the others. The environment is always more complex than the systems; it has more elements and relations. The systems get to observe their environment and try to reduce its complexities by selecting the aspects (elements and relations) that the system considers relevant for its autopoiesis. Systems do not have the "requisite variety" to relate each element from the environment to an element of the system. In other words, it is impossible for the system to map and represent all elements and relations of the environment. Because of that, systems have to make selections, reducing the complexity of the environment the system has to deal with. In this process, progressively, the system also becomes more complex, refining and developing new selections. But the system's complexity has to be controlled or even reduced to avoid overburdening the communicative operations of the system and its capacity to coordinate its own elements.

Systems' self-reference

As briefly mentioned in the discussions about health systems thinking (HST) in Chapters 4 and 5, HST says that systems are capable of self-organizing. Surely self-organizing needs to be understood as a broader attribute involving related capabilities such self-observation, self-description and so on, all included in the self-reference frame, which nevertheless, HST has not delved into. In contrast, systems theory tries to unravel the self-reference conundrum. The conceptualization of self-reference requires the confluence of a number of interrelated concepts, such as autopoiesis, operational closure, observation, selection and communications. Considering that a system can only carry out its reproduction internally, and the reproduction entails reproduction of consistent, connected, recursive and meaningful communications, a system needs to distinguish, recognize and validate communications belonging to it, separating them from the others. Validation of communications cannot come from the outside, therefore self-reference needs to continuously operate with the distinction system/environment. Self-reference makes possible the identification of meanings that make sense and therefore can communicatively be reproduced. Self-reference is defined in contrast with hetero-reference, as two sides of a distinction. However, autopoietic self-reference does not require the system to have an exhaustive, complete self-description and description of its environment. For the self-reference, it is enough that the system has identities and recognizes its limits; in other words, the system should be able to distinguish what belongs to it and what doesn't. This is done with the deployment of the recognized semantic codes and the symbols and signifiers the system operates with. Mistakes may happen, but the system has safeguards to keep its self-reference attuned, updated and, when necessary, corrected. Furthermore, the system has to deal with the paradoxical nature of self-reference, where referring to itself is referring to itself referring to itself and so on; this can go on to infinity. To halt the paradoxical eternal loop, self-reference has to stop the recurrence by electing an identity of the self, which can establish that no further exploration is required; the paradox is then halted and temporally solved. The patient needs to be treated and the discussion about the distinction between health/illness should stop; the system knows which side it has to pay attention to without getting entangled in self-reflection on its self-reference. The construction of identity is therefore a crucial step for the system and its capacity for self-observation, self-description and self-organizing. For identity construction, the system/environment distinction plays the fundamental role; what does not belong to the system belongs to the environment. Anyhow, and this adds complexity to the self-reference model, while the system may need the causalities inherent to the environment to stop the paradoxical tautology of self-reference, it relies on its internal representation of the environment as "interrupters of interdependencies". In Luhmann's (2015, p. 99) words,[1] "the system de-symmetrizes itself". In other words, to stop the tautological risks of its own self-referred loops, the system creates an asymmetry, internally referring back to the representations of the environment it created itself, recognizing the inherent causalities of the environment (the diseases and their causes), preserving in the process its operational closure and autopoiesis. In very simple terms, the health system not only treats the diseases created by it, but also treats illnesses according to orders of causalities the system can observe in the environment (the body of the patients).

Structural coupling of communication and consciousness

Luhmann refers to the independent autopoiesis of communication and consciousness and at the same time the fundamental role that one plays for the other. There would not be communication without consciousness and vice versa (at least for consciousness as we know it). But they reproduce independently, considering that only utterances link to utterances in the medium of communications and thoughts to other thoughts in the consciousness medium. What Alter communicates to Ego is not a copy of Alter's thoughts. The process of attaching content to utterances goes through selections of what it is possible to say, regardless of how far or close the results are to the meanings Alter has in his mind. On the other hand, the perceptions by Ego of the utterances made by Alter are further decoded with the selections Ego deploys in her own mind, whether or not she communicates about them. Ego's thoughts are not a copy of Alter's thoughts transferred by communication. In this sense, Luhmann speaks of an *orthogonal* relation between communication and consciousness. Their coupling do not eliminate their autonomy; precisely the opposite, coupling rather needs their independent autonomous performances.

A.2   Power and the political system

In the application of his Social System Theory to the political system, Niklas Luhmann developed an original conceptualization of power. In fact he used the same term and expanded the concept Talcott Parsons had established of power as a *symbolically generalized medium of communication*. This terminology

---

[1]   N. Luhmann (2015), *Sociedad y sistema: la ambición de la teoria*, ed. Paidós, Barcelona.

has crucial importance for understanding power and for research programmes based on it. The SGMC of power has a number of characteristics we discuss in this section before addressing the political system.

Power

To start with, a definition of medium and form is useful. A medium keeps loose connections among its elements while a form emerges within the medium by tightly connecting some of the components of the medium. A medium cannot be perceived in itself; it is known through forms by which it becomes recognizable. Forms are therefore perceivable by observers, who are capable of using the necessary distinctions to recognize the forms. The medium is full potential while a form is the actualization of only some of those potentialities. A form does not exhaust the medium, which, maintaining the loose connection between its elements, makes permanently possible the emergence of new forms. On the contrary, a form, in having its elements firmly connected, has little flexibility and can expire, be replaced or destroyed.[2] As an example, the medium of water can take a possibly infinite number of forms, depending on variables affecting the shape in which it is perceived. The medium of power takes form in the decisions communicated by the power-holders, for instance resolutions, decrees, orders, commands, regulations, policies, instructions and so on. The user of the medium makes the forms appear and makes them potentially communicable.

As a medium, power is unbounded potentiality where power communications are forms. To avoid the tautology, it can be explained that power communications involve asymmetrical exchange between Alter (the power-holder) and Ego (the power-subject), where Ego is led to take actions according to Alter's determinations, whether in agreement or not with Ego's wishes. While Alter has a range of options to select from, Ego is left with the one indicated by Alter. That in itself configures a specific order of communication, where Alter reduces uncertainties transferred to Ego, and by doing so also reduces the complexities faced by Ego. This model of communicative interaction is made possible by the acceptance on both sides of the inherent asymmetry, made communicatively possible by the use of a SGMC. By communicating through the

---

2   Luhmann addresses the conceptualization of medium and form in several books. However, concise explanation can be found in chapter 2, section 1, "Médium y forma" in Luhmann (2007, p. 145).

SGMC of power, Alter make their position recognizable by Ego, using the symbols that confers authenticity and legitimacy to the communication. The mad man in the psychiatric hospital impersonating Napoleon, giving orders in the ward, will not be recognized as issuing authentic and legitimate communications through the power medium. Even if he forms perfectly clear sentences, the power medium-coded symbols, recognizable by the recipient of the messages, will be missing.

The medium does not dictate the specific form the communication must take, but will convey with the communication a "stamp of validity", so to speak, certifying the propriety of the communication. The voice and the signature of the president, the privileged use of specific flags and emblems, the sequence of movements and speeches in rituals of power, the occupation of places in ministerial cabinet meetings, the channels and timing of official announcements, the ultimate discretion in selections of texts and communications, are just a few examples of symbolic representations and signifiers added to the utterances and content of communications assured by the power medium. The effectiveness of power medium comes from the motivation it elicits in Ego to follow the rulings, as well as in Alter, to issuing them.

In other words, the medium allows the form of power relations to take shape. As mentioned, in power relations the two sides recognize the medium in which they are communicating; therefore both acknowledge who exerts it for making decisions and who follows what is decided. Power is only present when the behaviour of the participants is ascribed to the symbolic code describing the situation as one of power. The medium does not have an ontological independent existence without the relations whereby it emerges (without the forms where it is manifested).

Power is exercised through communication

By being a medium of communications, power must be exercised by communications and only communications.[3] However, communications through this medium also have the characteristic of any communication: double contingency. Double contingency means that the two sides are aware that the communications involve selections on both sides and therefore messages are contingent (neither necessary nor impossible) and can be different. However, by the use of SGMC, the likelihood of acceptance and compliance increases.

---

3   See power as a medium of communication in Luhmann (2017b).

Like the communications expressing and sustaining them, power relations are contingent, repeating, they could be different; those involved could even occupy opposite positions. By being contingent, power relations are not based on fundamentals, i.e. transcendental or essential natural or sacred orders (even when they are justified as such), and they set the conditions of the exercises, with the permanent characteristic prospect of changeability of medium of communications. In other words, the medium does not prescribe beforehand who should be on which side of the power relation.

Of particular relevance, power-holders always have at their disposal the possibility of using negative sanctions including violence. But, by using violence the power-holder destroys the double contingency and the possibility of achieving the desired results through communicatively achieved compliance. Violence is therefore the failure of power as a medium of communication and shared symbolic code. Within the limits of the medium, a power-holder can go as far as threatening a violent act (issuing negative sanctions), which will affect the probability of subsequent communicative interlacing between Alter and Ego, but still preserves the communicative potential of the medium.

In Luhmann's view, violence is an alternative that both power-holders and power-subjects alike want to avoid. However, resorting to violence is never completely ruled out and remains a permanent possibility within political systems. In short, violence is a source of power precisely when it is not used.

In its differentiation in the society, the political system acquires the monopoly of the use of violent means and also has the prerogative to use power as a medium of communication. However, within societies, organizations also resort to use of the medium of power in its internal dealings. The symbols used are of a different nature and, given the close proximity between power-holders and power-subjects within the organizations, the exercise of power acquires specific characteristics and dynamics. Nevertheless, inside organizations, power is also exercised by communications (it could not be otherwise). But power-subjects have more decisive influence and participation in decisions and can mobilize counter-power of significant relevance, without breaking the asymmetry between power-holders and power-subjects. The destruction of the asymmetry would represent the collapse of the organization.

Power is necessary and also a risk for society

In Luhmann's words "Power is a universal factor of the life world and for societal existence" (Luhmann 2017b, p. 197). Power reduces complexities in societies structured by language and communication. This is the case because communication alone, with double contingencies, keeps open the chances of disadvantageous outcomes for both sides, with uncertainties prevailing throughout the processes of exchange and interaction. Power communication instead orientates the interlacing of the communications to a common outcome which, even not being Ego's favoured option, decreases uncertainties and therefore complexities. By communicating decisions through the power medium, Alter absorbs uncertainties, facilitating the subsequent interlacing.

In Luhmann's views, the power medium is an evolutionary achievement, a stage that allows society itself to reach higher levels of complexity in its internal differentiation. Once political systems are constituted and established as differentiated systems, with the prerogative of using the power medium (and monopoly of violence), all other function systems evolve in their own domains. Therefore, centralization of political power in the political system concurs with societal differentiation and autonomy of all other social systems. In this sense, political power centralized in the political system implies the recognition that there is also power outside the political system, which should remain operational within the systems and organizations using it, but should also remain depoliticized, unable to issue collectively binding decisions to be enforced upon the whole society. The challenge for societies that achieved differentiation of social systems is the preservation of both the monopoly of political power by the political system together with the existence of depoliticized power outside the political system.

The risk for systems-differentiated societies is the coexistence of political power held by the political system with uses of power communications by diverse social systems in their internal dealings. But not only that, the risk of misuse and abuse of political power is not curtailed by societies' fundamental communicativeness; communication and the use of SGMC do not rule out those possibilities; additional structures are needed.

The establishment of the legal system (a distinct, operationally closed and autonomous social system with its own binary code), and the exercise of political power through the medium of law, brings about what Luhmann calls the double coding of the power code into lawful power and unlawful power. The political system puts itself under the constraints of legality (so called "rule of law"), which nevertheless the twentieth century history has proved to be far from a perfect solution. In conclusion, the risks faced by the exercise of power in societies that underwent the differentiation in social function system streams from two sides: the risk of abuse of political powers and the risk of rendering political power too weak in face of the diversion of power away from the political system and dispersion among other function systems.

Exercise of power in organizations

Briefly recapitulating, Luhmann's social systems theory describes three types of autopoietic, operationally closed, communication-based social system: *function systems, organizations* and *interactions*.[4] The characteristics of organization and interaction can be explained as follows (see Chapter 7). *Organizations*[5] are constituted by two main aspects: 1) *membership*, by which only selected individuals can be considered members and participate in the organization; 2) *decisions*, which, as a specific type of communications (communicating actions to be taken), play a central role for the autopoiesis of the organization.[6] The life inside organizations consists in continuous communications of decisions among its members (with the related actions taking place accordingly). *Interactions* are social systems based on face-to-face contact between two or more people, where physical presence at the moment the communication takes place (including the use of any electronic media) is essential. Once the communication ends, the interaction system also ends.

Specifically in relation to power as medium, as mentioned previously, organizations do not have the same attributes of political power, but have specific functionalities that assure organization's operations and reproduction. In organizations, the emergence of power hierarchies and counter-power by power-subjects are of particular relevance. Reduction of complexities in organizations' internal communications involves the release of the power-holders from making all the decisions, having power-subjects empowered at their levels to make independent decisions in their respective fields of activities. At different points in the hierarchical chains, decisions are made without the participation of higher power-holders, whose expectations are already known and complied with without their involvement.

This use of power medium by mid-level subjects nevertheless creates the possibility of what Luhmann calls "countervailing power", also called "informal

---

4   For a comprehensive introduction of Luhmann's theory in the field of organization studies, see D. Seidl and H. Mormann (2014).
5   See book edited by Seidl and May for the several discussions applying Luhmann's concepts to organizational studies.
6   See *Organization and Decision* (Luhmann 2018).

power", that might in some respects become stronger than the power of the power-holder at the top. However, the full subversion and transformation of power-subjects into power-holders inside an organization would lead to its collapse. Power-holders know that by being granted a certain level of autonomy, power-subjects reduce the complexities faced by the power-holders themselves, but also know that there are limits to it. In short, the exercise of power inside organizations has a different outlook in comparison to political power exerted by the political system.

Political system

Luhmann's theory characterizes the function systems, and the political systems among them, with autopoietic drive under operational closure and dedicated use of specific binary codes. However, the political system has a number of specific features and structures.

The political system communicates within itself

The political system has three differentiated internal sub-systems, which communicate among themselves.[7] Before explaining the internal architecture, it is relevant to clarify Luhmann's understanding that the political system's communications are orientated towards autopoietic self-legitimation. The system strives to preserve and reproduce communications ascertaining its own legitimacy. In line with the theoretical notion of systems' closure, legitimation can only be self-legitimation, because no system can legitimate another. This might be a controversial and difficult point of the theory. In other words, the political system's priority and main concern is with its own legitimacy, which is assured and reproduced in its internal communications.

The three structural components of the political system are: administration, politics and the public, operating though as a unit. In Luhmann's words, "Administration means thereby the totality of institutions that creates binding decisions pursuant to political viewpoints and political mandate". "Politics sets

---

7   For a comprehensive discussion of the political and legal systems in Luhmann, see M. King and C. Thornhill (2003). From Luhmann himself, see Luhmann (1990), *Political Theory in the Welfare State*, Luhmann (2017b), *Trust and Power* and Luhmann (2014), *Sociología Política*.

boundaries and priorities for administrative decisions." "The Public participates through elections and other expressions of opinion" (Luhmann 1990, p. 48). This conceptual architecture does not neatly overlap with usual notion of separation of executive, legislative and judiciary powers of modern democracies.

As pointed out by King and Thornhill (2003, p. 86), "high-level decision (politics) and the departments of government (administration) which organize into generally acceptable media (laws, regulations, codes of practices, guidelines, and so on), Luhmann's schematic differentiation of politics hinges on a re-characterization of the executive as politics and on a re-characterization of the legislature as administration".

Thus constituted, the political system observes the environment it created within that system. That is the condition whereby collectively binding decisions are produced, which all other systems in the society must observe, for the sake of their own individual autopoiesis. All function systems, organizations and individuals (psychic systems) are "irritated" (condition for systems coupling) by the deliberations emanating from the political system.

On the other hand, by observing and being "irritated" by its environment, where the other function systems, organizations and population in general are, the political sub-systems bring in for internal elaboration, and concurrent exchanges among its divisions, the themes and subjects that require political attention and decision for the establishment of collectively binding rules. This preserves the operational closure of the system and simultaneously the reliability of the power medium of communication and its binary code. Legitimation is in fact constructed in the internal works of the system, in the continuous validation (or rejection) of the relevance of the topics, the need for ruling, and the acceptability of the rules.

This snapshot is a very short summary of a rather complex theoretical construction, to which Luhmann dedicated specific books. Luhmann uses the same theoretical construct of internal differentiation inside a function system for his analysis of the economic and legal system; the theoretical expediency allows for unification of a diversity of sub-functions under the same processes of internal self-organization and self-regulation.[8]

---

8   See the conceptualization of the internal differentiation of the political system in section 5, "Politics as a Self-Referential System", of chapter 2 in Luhmann (1990). For the description of the internal differentiation in the Economic System, see chapter 3, "El Mercado como entorno interno del sistema económico" in Luhmann (2017a).

Health system and the political system

This final point concerns the relationship between the health system and the political system and how health policies fit into the proposed scheme. Health policies approved and enacted by the political system are examples of "collectively binding decisions" that are prerogatives of the political system. No single health institution would be able to issue a policy that could be enforced across all health services delivery organizations, given the diverse nature of the organizations and non-existence of a single body to which all would be subordinated. This is the context found in the large majority of countries, with perhaps just a few exceptions, where the Ministry of Health is the sole provider of health services of all types.

Nevertheless, the political system is empowered to make decisions that can affect all under its political jurisdiction. That is one of the main features of the relationship between health and political systems, acknowledging the political power prerogatives the health system cannot have. Likewise, in the differentiation of the functional systems, the political system cannot obviously make diagnostics or deliver treatments, or even elaborate health risk assessment of populations. The political system cannot communicate on health matters with the authority and legitimacy that only the health system can.

The political system can be "irritated" on health matters (through the health system's public health interface or through the communications internal to the political system that reflect, for instance, constituencies' expectations and political promises and pressures). Irritation may reach a level that forces the political system to act in the name of the gathering expectations and the calls for legitimation constantly raised internally in the political system.

The Ministry of Health is a member of the political system, raising issues and responding when it is demanded; it is one of the voices communicating interests and expectations on health-related matters inside the political system, as members of the public (as noted above, a specific sub-system of the political system) also can do.

While political processes may unfold inside the political system, the life (communications) inside the health system go on independently, with patients being identified and treated continuously. On the health system's side, the configuration is of a vast universe of never-ending health communications over which the political system can have no determination. Health communications interlace subsequent communications, selecting and reproducing the means of reproducing the communications, in recurrent self-observation processes, which are of very high complexity for external observers. To large extent, the political system is almost entirely an external observer of the health system, if it were not for the bridges that the Ministry of Health builds, through its public health division.

Although the political system remains with the monopoly of political power and the capability of enacting collectively binding decisions, that cannot affect the autopoietic driving function of the health system. The political system can have only a very limited impact on the complexity the health system itself maintains and carries on with.

Conclusion

The unpacking and clarification of the structural complexities of the interwoven wealth of concepts found in Luhmann's work on political systems is a task that requires many pages. What has been attempted here nevertheless is only a summary presentation of key ideas found throughout several of his books. The purpose has been to explain the concepts and how they are interlinked in the theoretical architecture. The text is far from exhaustive regarding the thinking in Luhmann's social systems theory, and does not reflect the works that discuss and criticize Luhmann's work from the perspective of other theoretical approaches on power and politics.[9] The main intention was to explain the power theory built on the fundamental notion of communication in the functioning of the political system, describing its interlinks with other function systems, specifically the health social system.

---

9   For discussions of Luhmann's views from other perspectives, some key references are M. King and C. Thornhill (2003), with a comprehensive discussion of Luhmann's critics particularly for his self-referred "anti-humanism" and superficial criticism of his alleged conservatism. The two books by H. Moeller (2005 and 2012) and the book by W. Rasch (2000) present valuable discussions of the philosophical basis of Luhmann's work and the main currents such as post-modernism, Derrida, Lyotard, Foucault, Habermas, as well as previous philosophical thoughts, from Kant and Hegel up to Husserl and Heidegger. H. Moeller (2005) and D. Seidl and K. Helg (2006) also provide concise useful glossaries of key terms of the theory.

Social Sciences

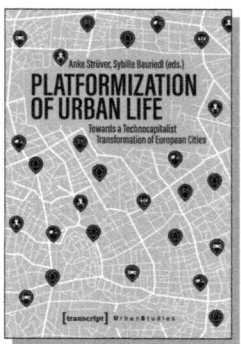

Anke Strüver, Sybille Bauriedl (eds.)
Platformization of Urban Life
Towards a Technocapitalist Transformation
of European Cities

September 2022, 304 p., pb.
29,50 € (DE), 978-3-8376-5964-1
E-Book: available as free open access publication
PDF: ISBN 978-3-8394-5964-5

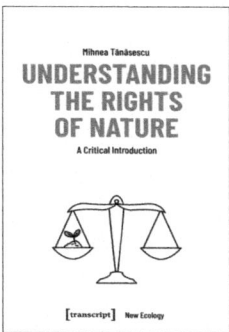

Mihnea Tanasescu
Understanding the Rights of Nature
A Critical Introduction

February 2022, 168 p., pb.
40,00 € (DE), 978-3-8376-5431-8
E-Book: available as free open access publication
PDF: ISBN 978-3-8394-5431-2

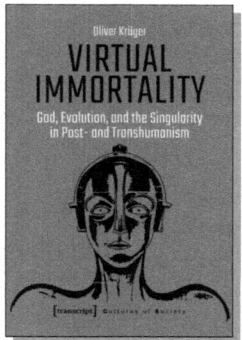

Oliver Krüger
**Virtual Immortality –
God, Evolution, and the Singularity
in Post- and Transhumanism**

2021, 356 p., pb., ill.
35,00 € (DE), 978-3-8376-5059-4
E-Book:
PDF: 34,99 € (DE), ISBN 978-3-8394-5059-8

**All print, e-book and open access versions of the titles in our list
are available in our online shop www.transcript-publishing.com**

Social Sciences

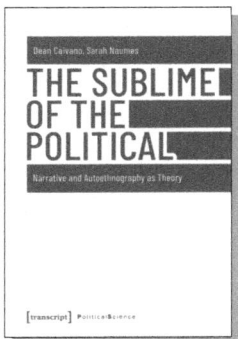

Dean Caivano, Sarah Naumes
The Sublime of the Political
Narrative and Autoethnography as Theory

2021, 162 p., hardcover
100,00 € (DE), 978-3-8376-4772-3
E-Book:
PDF: 99,99 € (DE), ISBN 978-3-8394-4772-7

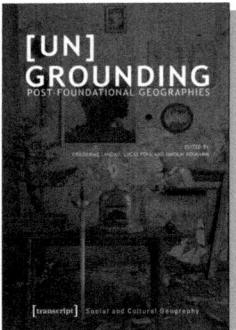

Friederike Landau, Lucas Pohl, Nikolai Roskamm (eds.)
[Un]Grounding
Post-Foundational Geographies

2021, 348 p., pb., col. ill.
50,00 € (DE), 978-3-8376-5073-0
E-Book:
PDF: 49,99 € (DE), ISBN 978-3-8394-5073-4

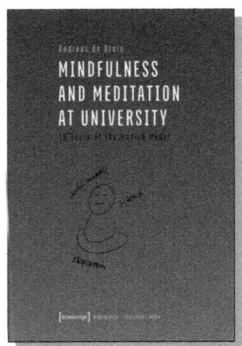

Andreas de Bruin
Mindfulness and Meditation at University
10 Years of the Munich Model

2021, 216 p., pb.
25,00 € (DE), 978-3-8376-5696-1
E-Book: available as free open access publication
PDF: ISBN 978-3-8394-5696-5

All print, e-book and open access versions of the titles in our list are available in our online shop www.transcript-publishing.com